Freedom
from
ASTHMA

Freedom
from
ASTHMA

THE REVOLUTIONARY
5-Day TREATMENT
FOR HEALING ASTHMA
WITH THE BREATH CONNECTION® PROGRAM

Alexander Stalmatski
with Brigid McConville

Foreword by Dr. Konstantin Buteyko

Three Rivers Press
New York

The information given in this book is intended for general guidance and is not a sub-stitute for individual diagnosis or treatment by a qualified practitioner or medical doc-tor. Always consult a medical doctor and qualified practitioner before embarking on any treatment. The reader is strongly advised not to attempt self-treatment for any seri-ous or long-term complaint without consulting a medical doctor or qualified practi-tioner. Neither the author, the publishers, nor the Hale Clinic can be held responsible for any adverse reaction to the recommendations contained in this book, which are fol-lowed entirely at the reader's own risk.

All bona fide Breath Connection practitioners offer a money-back guarantee of sub-stantial improvement for every patient they have agreed to treat, no matter what the complaint.

Published by Three Rivers Press, 201 East 50th Street, New York, New York 10022. Member of the Crown Publishing Group.

Originally published in Great Britain in 1997 by Kyle Cathie Limited.

Random House, Inc. New York, Toronto, London, Sydney, Auckland
www.randomhouse.com
Three Rivers Press is a registered trademark of Random House, Inc.

Printed in the United States of America

Design by Leonard Henderson

Library of Congress Cataloging-in-Publication Data
Stalmatski, Alexander.
    Freedom from asthma : the revolutionary five-day treatment for
healing asthma / by Alexander Stalmatski, with Brigid McConville ;
with a foreword by Konstantin Buteyko.
    Includes bibliographical references and index.
    1. Asthma—Alternative treatment.   2. Asthma—Exercise therapy.
3. Breathing exercises.   4. Carbon dioxide—Physiological effect.
I. McConville, Brigid.   II. Title.
RC591.S72   1999
616.2'3806—dc21   98-37223

ISBN 0-609-80369-7

10 9 8 7 6 5 4 3 2 1
First American Edition

ACKNOWLEDGMENTS

The author and publishers wish to thank Tess Graham and all the other Buteyko patients who shared their experiences. The case history on Marjorie Curtis on pages 68–69 is adapted from an article that appeared in the *Buteyko Breathers' Bulletin* and is reproduced courtesy of the Buteyko Supporters' Association in Australia.

CONTENTS

FOREWORD

On October 7, 1952, I happened to be the first scientist in the world to discover the major cause of a number of diseases of the respiratory, hormonal, cardiovascular, and nervous systems, which were incurable by modern medicine. Forty-five years of scientific research and practical work on my method (known in the West as the Breath Connection or the Buteyko Method) allow me to claim that this drug-free process is perfectly safe and immeasurably more effective than traditional drug treatment of many chronic disorders—especially asthma. Scientific trials of my method in the treatment of asthma (in Russia in 1968 and 1981 and in Australia from 1994 to 1995) showed results unseen in the whole of medical history and proved the accuracy of the observations I first made forty-five years ago.

While my method is very popular in Russia, Australia, and New Zealand, in Europe and North America it is relatively new and largely unknown—yet. Therefore I am glad that this book—written by one of my best pupils and practitioners, Sasha Stalmatski—will inform readers of my discovery. I hope that in time a Buteyko practitioner will be found in every corner of the globe and my treatment will be available to all.

I bless this book and hope that it will change the lives of many sufferers.

Dr. Konstantin Buteyko
Professor of Medicine
Moscow
July 1997

1

DR. BUTEYKO AND HIS REVOLUTIONARY TREATMENT FOR ASTHMA

"Who is this Dr. Buteyko?" people often ask me. "I have never heard of him. And why—if it is so good—is his method not more widely recognized?"

I reply that Dr. Buteyko is a Russian and as well known in Russia as the Queen Mother is in Britain. But just as very few people in Russia have ever heard of the Queen Mother, very few people in Britain—or anywhere else in the Western world—have yet heard of Dr. Buteyko.

There are complex historical and political reasons, too, for Dr. Buteyko being relatively unknown in the West. For many years his mail was intercepted, his telephone was bugged, and his work was classified as a "state secret." He was not free to travel or to talk about his ideas in the West. Buteyko is not as famous as Andrey Sakharov or Alexandr

Solzhenitsyn, but he had the weight of the Russian medical establishment against him. He suffered ridicule in his own country for his ideas, and at one point the state tried to incarcerate him in a mental hospital. Fortunately he was saved by a senior member of the Communist Party, whom he had treated successfully.

Nonetheless Dr. Buteyko made many discoveries, which turned the whole range of medical treatments on its head. It was some forty-five years ago when, as a young intern working in a hospital for terminally ill patients, he observed that an increase in breathing was an indicator of approaching death. He realized that he could predict the time of death by monitoring patients' breathing patterns and that deepening breathing was linked to a wide range of diseases and chronic conditions.

Over the years Buteyko studied hundreds of patients and developed the theory that much ill health is the result of the body's defense mechanisms trying to compensate for lack of carbon dioxide. Deep breathing, he argued, was not just a symptom but a cause of illnesses ranging from cardiac problems to breathing disorders.

He not only discovered that overbreathing, or hyperventilation, is the cause of asthma; he also developed a method of measuring breathing and the connections between carbon dioxide, hyperventilation, and bronchospasm—the involuntary contraction of the bronchial (lung) tubes which is part of the cause of an asthma attack.

He explained many phenomena that medicine had been unable to understand for hundreds of years—such as exercise-induced asthma, nocturnal asthma, emotional asthma, and the links between asthma, stress, and infections. Dr. Buteyko has also explained why the modern medical concept of asthma treatment is problematic at best and has pointed out the detrimental effects of asthma drugs, past and present. He has explained why steroids (in the correct quantities) can help asthmatics—and (in overdose) can also harm or prove fatal to them.

In addition, Dr. Buteyko has shown the connections between overbreathing and a whole host of other complaints, including allergy, anxiety, panic attacks, nasal problems, eczema, headaches, emphysema, bronchitis, and hay fever. He has explained why people die from asthma and how this can be prevented.

His method of retraining breathing involves a series of exercises designed to restore normal breathing patterns by retraining the body's respiratory center in the brain. This, in a nutshell, is the program known as the Breath Connection, modeled on Buteyko's treatment of respiratory diseases. It can provide an effective self-management treatment not only for asthma but for allergies, insomnia, bronchitis, anxiety, migraines, high blood pressure, and hemorrhoids—to name a few. Even the worldwide problem of blocked noses and snoring can benefit from the Breath Connection!

BUTEYKO ON TRIAL

The Breath Connection is not proclaimed as a success by asthma experts because it is a drug-free treatment, and as such it poses a serious threat to the profits of drug companies and pharmacists around the world, as well as to the reputations of doctors, hospitals, and academics everywhere.

An important aspect of the comparatively low profile of the Breath Connection in the Western world has been the extreme reluctance of asthma "specialists" to consider the evidence of its effectiveness. The initial reaction of the Australian

Asthma Foundation was to issue a special warning that the Breath Connection was dangerous. Then it admitted that for every successful Breath Connection treatment of asthma, there is one case which is not successful—suggesting that the Breath Connection has a 50 percent success rate! Not bad for something that has been written off as dangerous!

In 1993 the Australian Asthma Foundation agreed to observe a workshop in Adelaide, on the condition that the results of their observations remain confidential. In this workshop of thirty-six participants, including people suffering from severe asthma and emphysema, everybody derived some benefit from the Breath Connection (including two observers, one of whom got rid of a blocked-nose problem, while the other learned how to overcome and then prevent her own asthma attacks).

The Australian Asthma Campaign observed another Breath Connection workshop in Melbourne, during May 1994. Data from this workshop was analyzed by Professor Charles Mitchell, an internationally respected asthma specialist, who in October 1994 advised that as a result of the Breath Connection, 75 percent of the workshop's participants reported that their asthma symptoms occurred less frequently, and 90 percent had been able to reduce their medication. Professor Mitchell also sent three of his severely asthmatic patients to learn the Breath Connection and reported that they derived great benefit from this treatment within one week.

In 1994 an eight-month scientific trial was at last set up by the Australian Asthma Foundation after intense pressure from the public and the media to investigate the Breath Connection. It followed a period of many years during which asthma specialists had tried to ignore or discredit the Breath Connection.

This trial was conducted at the Mater Hospital, Brisbane,

from 1994 to 1995 (see Appendix 3, page 161). The result was a 90 percent reduction in the use of bronchodilators and a 49 percent reduction in the use of steroids by participants in the trial. The country's leading medical magazine, *Australian Doctor*, published two articles on the trial entitled "Doctors Gasp at Buteyko [The Breath Connection's] Success" and "Buteyko Lowers Need for Drugs."

Disappointingly, at the time of writing this new edition, these entirely positive results have yet to be communicated to the public by the Australian Asthma Foundation. It seems that some doctors are willing to prescribe asthma drugs without understanding fully how they work, but they are not willing to try the Breath Connection—because they don't understand fully how it works.

Fortunately many Australians have discovered for themselves that the Breath Connection is effective, and the network of Breath Connection teachers and supporters is growing fast, but the same story of suspicion and reluctance to accept the success of Breath Connection treatments is being repeated in Britain and the United States.

In Australia and New Zealand it is the media (as well as the people who have been successfully treated by the Breath Connection) who have spread the news that now there is a treatment which can stop asthma once and for all. And again, this pattern is beginning to take hold in Britain, where reputable journals have called for asthma specialists not to dismiss a potential cure for asthma out of hand.

IS THE BREATH CONNECTION A CURE?

What I can say very clearly is that the Breath Connection is the best-known route to a cure. After two or three days of treatment, you will be able to reduce your medication by 40 to 50 percent—because of the improvement in your condition. After a few more days, you should be able to reduce your medication by 80 to 100 percent. After a few weeks (for children), or a few months (for severe, chronic asthmatics), you will be able to live without medications and without asthma attacks.

This is the best method of asthma management ever discovered. And what a contrast to modern medicine, which leads asthmatics to a dead end of long-term treatment without solving the problem.

The Breath Connection is a discovery that could enable millions of people the world over to protect themselves against one of the most insidious epidemics of our time. Not AIDS, but asthma. While doctors and patients are fighting a losing battle against this rampant disease, desperately treating the symptoms because they do not know the cause, the observations of a Russian medical scientist, Dr. Konstantin Buteyko, will help us not only to understand asthma but to prevent it.

What has come to be known as the Breath Connection is simply a course of exercises to retrain our breathing patterns, and it is an effective drug-free treatment for asthma as well as for some 150 other disorders.

ASTHMA IS A BREATHING DISORDER

In our culture there is a widespread assumption that deep breathing is good for us because it increases our oxygen intake. In fact the reverse is true: The more you breathe, the less oxygen actually gets to the cells of your body.

This is because the air around you contains a much smaller proportion of carbon dioxide than your own body.

Carbon dioxide is essential for your body's uptake of oxygen. Breathing too much, or overbreathing, results in a deficit of carbon dioxide, which reduces the level of oxygen in your blood and tissues—affecting the function of every system in your body. Retrain your breathing, and you will cure your asthma. It is as simple as that.

MAD ENOUGH TO BE BRILLIANT?

Dr. Buteyko's theory about overbreathing overturns many of the assumptions of modern medicine (and modern drug therapy). Some people reading this book may shake their heads and say, "That Dr. Buteyko must be mad! Everyone knows that it is not like that!"

However, the history of medicine shows that new discoveries have often been condemned as "mad." Take the Hungarian obstetrician and surgeon Ignaz Semmelweis, who in 1846 discovered the causes of sepsis—the invasion of the body by "rotting" bacteria. In the 1890s, an average of thirteen women a day died in England and Wales of an infection known as "childbed fever," after giving birth. Today, largely thanks to our knowledge of antiseptics, the mortality rate for this disease has plummeted to one maternal death a week—despite the fact that twice as many women are giving birth.

Semmelweis put forward a theory that doctors should wash their hands before delivering babies and before performing surgery. His "mad" idea earned him ridicule, rejection, and, ultimately, confinement in a lunatic asylum, where he died. Sadly another half century would pass before his emphasis on hand washing was widely adopted by doctors.

It was Niels Bohr, the founder of nuclear physics, who said that for a discovery to be brilliant it had to be crazy. So when

people say that Dr. Buteyko must be mad, it is worth consid-
ering whether his ideas are mad enough to be truly brilliant.
Certainly his fundamental and far-reaching theory has been
met with skepticism (at the very least) by many modern doctors and asthma specialists.

2

WHAT IS ASTHMA?

ASTHMA ON THE RISE

We've known about the disease we now call asthma for four thousand years, but modern medicine has so far failed to discover its causes—or to find a cure. Modern medical treatments are unsatisfactory, while doctors have little idea of how to prevent this disease. Yet statistics show a dramatic increase in asthma in the Western world, painting a very worrisome picture.

Asthma

- is the only disease in the Western world that is increasing to epidemic proportions;
- has for forty years defeated modern medicine's attempts to reduce the number of deaths it causes;
- has doubled its occurrence in children since the 1970s.

Surveys of U.K. schoolchildren conducted over the last ten years all point to the startling fact that in Britain one child in eight now has asthma. An even higher proportion of those surveyed—one in five—has suffered from wheezing at some time in childhood. There are *more than 15 million asthmatics in the United States*. Every year more than five thousand people die from asthma in the United States alone.

Unfortunately careful repeat studies point to a real increase in asthma. So why should this be? Various theories have been put forward to explain the rise in asthma, including air pollution, stress—and even the weather.

But while there is no doubt that pollution in our cities, particularly when combined with allergies, can trigger symptoms in people who already have asthma, there is no evidence that pollution creates more asthmatics. What's more, asthma is just as prevalent in the Scottish Highlands as it is in relatively smoggy urban areas.

So what about stress? Could this be causing increasing rates of asthma? I believe it is a fallacy that we are under more stress today than were our ancestors, whose daily struggles for survival were much more primal than ours. By contrast, we live relatively easy and protected lives. Of course stress can exacerbate asthma—whether you feel anger, depression, anxiety, joy, or excitement—but stress itself cannot create asthma in the first place.

Some people have suggested that if asthma can be influenced by psychological events, asthmatics ought to have a readily identifiable type of personality. Over the years asthmatics have been described in a number of unflattering ways, ranging from irritable and fearful to complaining and obsessively neurotic. But it strikes me as extremely unfair to blame a person who has a severe and frightening disease for being nervous and depressed, especially if you are going to treat them with drugs which will not eradicate their asthma.

As for the weather, in hot Israel, cold Canada, cool New Zealand, and warm Australia, people still suffer from asthma. In the United States, which has all sorts of weather, 5,500 people die from asthma every year. Of course, some people with asthma feel better or worse in certain types of weather, but they still have asthma. Today, asthma is on the increase all over the globe. What then is the reason or reasons for the phenomenal rise in its rates of occurrence in the modern world?

We have become obsessed with asthma. Doctors now try to diagnose it very early in children, often too early, so that illnesses previously called "wheezy bronchitis" are now labeled asthma and treated accordingly. When you visit your doctor because you have the flu or a cold, he or she may well put you on asthma medications—"just in case." You start taking them and then, after a while, you discover that you now need them. You think you have developed asthma!

Probably the country most obsessed with asthma is Australia, where one in four children and one in ten adults are already diagnosed as having the disease. By the year 2020, medical authorities expect that one Australian in two will have asthma, and in a sadly self-fulfilling prophecy, so far it looks as if they are going to make it!

TRYING TO MAKE SENSE OF ASTHMA: THE MEDICAL VIEW

Traditional medicine has viewed asthma as the lungs' over-reaction to an irritant or allergen. When the body senses a foreign or toxic substance, it launches an attack against the invader. In a defensive response to an invader, the lining of the respiratory passages becomes swollen and air does not easily pass through. Mucus develops to help protect the irritated tissue, but as it coats the tissue, it further blocks the airways. Nerves send signals to the muscles around the bronchial tubes, which cause them to constrict the airways even further.

TRIGGER FACTORS, BUT NOT THE CAUSE

There are thousands of factors that can trigger an asthma attack, but modern medicine isolates six main trigger factors (as opposed to causes of asthma).

- Exercise
- Viruses
- Infections
- Emotional factors such as stress
- Allergies
- Drugs

Asthma has been treated sometimes by prescribing dangerous medicines and steroids that open up the airways for a period of time. The symptoms of the disease are addressed, but there is no attempt to go to the root of the problem or to teach preventative measures for dealing with the asthma.

Traditionally, doctors have divided the disease into allergic (extrinsic) and nonallergic asthma. There are many people whose asthma is clearly triggered by allergic reactions, yet there are many others who have asthma attacks for a variety of reasons—some of them having to do with allergies, but some not.

There is also another group of asthma sufferers who have no allergic problems, and they have been classified as having "idiopathic" asthma. This sounds impressive, but in fact *idiopathic* just means that the disease is unique to the individual patient, or in other words, "We don't know the cause."

Misunderstanding of the nature of asthma by conventional medicine has produced a complex division of asthma into different types. If you wake up in the night unable to breathe you have nocturnal asthma; if walking upstairs makes you breathless you have exercise-induced asthma; if you get symptoms when you laugh it is emotional asthma— and so on for occupational asthma (from your job), environmental asthma (from pollution), aspirin asthma (from taking aspirin), and self-induced asthma (no doubt from crying about the injustice of having this confusing disease!).

All this reminds me of the classification of animals in ancient China. The Chinese view was that there were twelve types of animal: those belonging to the emperor, those which are small and jump, and so on, down to the final category, which comprised all animals not included in the previous groups!

However modern medicine tries to classify asthma, the clinical picture of an attack remains the same (see page 25), whether it is induced by laughing or crying or sex or ice cream. And yet there is still no consensus among doctors, scientists, and "asthma educators" about the causes of asthma, or even about the causes of these different types of asthma.

WHY MODERN MEDICAL TREATMENTS ARE UNSATISFACTORY

Some 90 percent of modern medical treatment for asthma involves prescription drugs. The other 10 percent consists of advice on how to take the drugs properly, how to avoid trigger factors such as dust mites, how to maintain your best "peak flow meter" readings (see page 119), and, sometimes, physiotherapy (see page 120). But in spite of these treatments, rates of asthma in the Western world are getting worse, not better. Meanwhile, many people with asthma are suffering side effects from drug treatments.

It is also difficult or impossible to avoid many of the common trigger factors—such as atmospheric pollution or emotional upheaval—while peak flow meter readings are strangely resistant to all efforts to improve them. And from a Breath Connection point of view, most physiotherapy only makes asthma worse.

The sad reality is that modern asthma treatments can go on for twenty, forty, even sixty years. Eventually dealing with asthma becomes a lifestyle, and asthma patients may well outlive their doctors, without ever finding a way to end the disease that dominates their lives.

The fundamental problem with modern medical treatments is that they treat the symptoms of asthma—such as wheezing, coughing, phlegm, and constriction of the airways—without tackling the cause. Yet in the words of Hippocrates two and a half thousand years ago, "Not knowing the cause, the doctor has no right to treat the disease."

Treating the cause of a disease is very different from treating the disease's symptoms. Let's take, for example, the story of the bubonic plague and its treatment. This disease used to "clean up" half of Europe rather as a winning poker player "cleans up" at the table. At the time, many people considered it to be God's punishment for sin and they treated themselves accordingly by going to church to pray (unless they were already infected, in which case they had to pray at home). They used other prophylactics, too, such as dressing in black and shouting, "The Black Death is coming!"

But that was about all that people could do until, in 1882, Robert Koch discovered the real cause of the plague. It was not a punishment from God after all, it was a bacillus called

Yersinia pestis. Once the cause of the plague was understood, the cure for it—through vaccination—could be found.

A NEW VIEW OF ASTHMA: THE BREATH CONNECTION

What makes the Breath Connection crucially different from modern medical treatments is that it recognizes that asthma is a breathing disorder; therefore it sets out to investigate and change our breathing patterns. Once we understand the cause of asthma, we can do something about stopping its occurrence. Once we eliminate the cause, the problem will disappear. If you can learn to normalize your breathing, you will not have asthma again, in spite of colds, playing sports, laughing, traveling, smoking, or making love. There is only one thing you must not do: You must not overbreathe, or hyperventilate. If you do, you are breaking one of nature's most important laws, and the asthma may return.

WHAT IS AN ASTHMA ATTACK?

An asthma attack happens when the tiny bronchial tubes in your lungs become narrowed or constricted, making it difficult to breathe.

This constriction of the airways is caused by a combination of three factors:

- Bronchospasm, when the muscle rings around the airways contract
- Swelling of the membranes of the airways so that the air spaces are narrowed
- An excess of mucus in the airways, secreted by the cells lining the bronchial tubes

An asthma attack is a vicious circle of hyperventilation, because as your airways narrow, spasm, and become blocked by mucus, you feel an increasing need to breathe deeply. You may panic, gasping desperately for air, as your body's three defense mechanisms work to make sure you don't increase your hyperventilation. The harder you try to breathe, the worse your asthma attack becomes—unless, using the Breath Connection, you learn to use techniques to bring your breathing under control.

ASTHMA—BREATHING DISORDER

Breathing is perhaps the most important function of our bodies. Every day we breathe in and out more than twenty thousand times. We can survive for weeks without food, quite a few days without sleep and water, but only a few minutes without breathing. Yet even as we approach the end of the twentieth century, most people's understanding of breathing is still very limited.

CARBON DIOXIDE IS NOT A WASTE GAS

Until the second half of the eighteenth century, physicians believed that air was drawn into the lungs for the purpose of cooling the blood. Then the French chemist Antoine Lavoisier came up with his theory that oxygen was the "gas of life"—as opposed to carbon dioxide, which was considered a waste gas that we breathe out. Hence, Lavoisier gave the name *oxygen* to what has since been thought of as the gas of life. By contrast, carbon dioxide, which was shown to kill mice at high

trachea

main bronchus

bronchiole

lung

inner wall with mucus-
secreting cells

inner wall swells and
the space within the
bronchiole narrows

smooth
muscle ring

mucus is secreted
and further
narrows the
airway

muscle rings
contract

normal bronchiole

**bronchiole during
asthma attack**

What happens during an asthma attack

concentrations, was believed to be a poisonous, or, at best, a waste gas. However, in a later experiment, baby mice were put in a container with pure oxygen, and as a result, this gas of life made them blind. For some reason, not many people know about this experiment.

The common, but false, assumption that after inhaling oxygen we exhale a waste gas called carbon dioxide (CO_2) has led to a fundamental misunderstanding of asthma. In fact, carbon dioxide is one of the most important chemical regulators of the human body, monitoring the activity of the heart, the blood vessels, and the respiratory system.

- The rate and depth of our breathing is regulated by the amount of carbon dioxide in our blood, as John Haldane discovered in 1905.
- When carbon dioxide is removed from the body in undue quantities by excessive artificial ventilation of the lungs, the heart and blood circulation gradually fail and death results, as Yale University professor Yandell Henderson discovered in 1909.

The level of oxygen in the room where you are reading this book is 20 percent—the normal level of this gas in our atmosphere. You would probably not notice if the oxygen level doubled or even tripled around you because our bodies are "blind" to higher levels of oxygen. And if the oxygen level dropped considerably, you would be unlikely to notice any difference in your breathing. Only if the level dropped below 15 percent—as it does at high altitudes—would you be aware of the difference.

Contrast the situation with carbon dioxide. Asthmatics have between 3.5 and 4.5 percent of carbon dioxide in their alveolar air. If this was to be decreased by as little as 0.1 percent, anyone—whether he or she was asthmatic or not—would develop dizziness, palpitations, wheezing, a blocked nose, or a mild asthma attack.

These figures indicate that our bodies are fifty times more sensitive to changes in the levels of carbon dioxide than they are to changes in oxygen levels. It follows that carbon dioxide is far more important to your body than oxygen. If asthmatics can normalize their carbon dioxide level by raising it to 5.5 or 6 percent, they can get rid of their asthma. Experiments have shown that a level of more than 10 percent carbon dioxide causes loss of consciousness, but there is never any need to increase carbon dioxide to such an extent, and the Breath Connection certainly does not involve raising carbon dioxide levels above normal.

The logical conclusion seemed to be that we should all inhale more of the gas of life in order to be healthy and also exhale more waste gas. Over the decades this idea has been promoted by physiotherapists, yoga teachers, doctors, sports coaches, army sergeants, and aerobics instructors. In the absence of even one scientific article to prove that deep breathing is good, it remains one of the great superstitions of the twentieth century.

However, there are hundreds of scientific studies that show that overbreathing causes a whole range of health problems, just as overeating and having high blood sugar, high blood pressure, or high blood cholesterol act as detriments to your health. For all essential aspects of health there are established norms, well known to the medical profession—except, strangely enough, breathing!

Actually, there *is* a norm for breathing, but few doctors know of it. This is not the peak flow measure used in conventional treatments for asthma, but a norm which depends (as the other norms do) on your age, height, gender, and size. It is called the "minute volume," and with the use of sophisticated equipment (available in some hospitals) it measures your lung ventilation in terms of the liters of air you breathe per minute.

A physiologically normal minute volume is between four and six liters of air per minute while you are at rest (less for children). People with asthma typically breathe two, three, or four times that amount; in other words, if you have asthma you are breathing enough for two, three, or four people. This is called hyperventilation, and, according to Buteyko, it is the major cause of asthma.

A PIONEERING STUDY OF BREATHING

One of history's great investigators into breathing was British physiologist John Haldane (1860–1936). He developed methods that enabled scientists to learn how much oxygen and carbon dioxide are contained in a person's blood and lungs at any time and how our bodies regulate breathing response to these substances. Haldane also studied the breathing process and the amounts of energy that our bodies use in order to breathe.

Haldane's work had so helped us to understand the fundamental principles of human breathing that by the mid-twentieth century it was established that oxygen passes into our bloodstreams through the thin membranes of the alveoli without having to be "pumped" by any other process. It was Haldane, too, who established the importance of the right quantities of carbon dioxide in our breathing by the techniques he invented of sampling the gas in the alveoli.

Haldane's book *Respiration* (1922), with its analysis of alveolar air, influenced many scientists—in particular, the medical student Konstantin Buteyko.

Ultimately Haldane became involved in secret research for the British navy, which involved studying the control of oxygen and carbon dioxide in damaged submarines. Many of his findings are still classified as top secret. Unfortunately he was not interested in asthma, which in his day was not considered a fatal disease. Yet his work helped us to understand that the process we call respiration is not just a matter of inhaling oxygen and exhaling carbon dioxide.

HOW WE BREATHE

When you breathe, air passes from your windpipe (trachea) into your two main airways (bronchi). From there it goes through the small bronchioles to the tiny air sacs (alveoli) where oxygen is absorbed into your bloodstream. But then, far from going directly to the cells of our bodies, it goes through a complex chemical process called respiration.

Most oxygen molecules are carried in the blood by the red blood cells (although 5 percent of it is dissolved in plasma, the colorless fluid that remains after red cells are filtered out of the blood). The material in red blood cells which grabs and holds oxygen molecules is called hemoglobin, which combines with oxygen to make a new molecule called oxyhemoglobin.

Once this oxygen-rich blood reaches the cells of the body that need it, the oxygen detaches itself from the red blood cells, to be used by the body's metabolism (the complex series of chemical reactions that transform fats, sugars, and proteins into energy). It is hemoglobin that makes it possible for your blood to carry the oxygen you need. Without it—if oxygen were only dissolved in plasma—your heart would

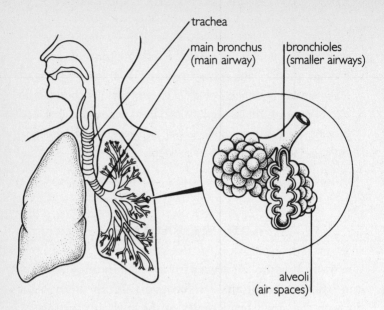

The structure of the lungs

have to pump about twenty-five times as fast to deliver enough oxygen to your body's cells.

Sometimes, however, hemoglobin can't release its oxygen to the body, and the heart starts pumping overtime. This is what happens to many asthmatics during an asthma attack: They feel a lack of oxygen, so they desperately try to take in air, perhaps opening the windows in an attempt to get more oxygen. Yet despite breathing rapidly, often through the mouth, it doesn't seem to help.

Why should this be? Surely—as we have been led to believe—deep breathing gives us more oxygen.

But this is the paradox that lies at the heart of understanding the Breath Connection: The truth is that when you overbreathe (i.e., breathe more than the physiological norm)

An oxygen molecule's journey to the bloodstream

you are actually getting less oxygen, not more. This is because our bodies need to maintain a certain level of carbon dioxide in the blood in order for our hemoglobin to release the oxygen we need.

When we overbreathe, we are upsetting the delicate balance between the carbon dioxide and oxygen in our bloodstreams that we need to maintain in order to make use of the oxygen in our body cells. Yes, we are breathing in more oxygen, but we are also breathing out more carbon dioxide, and without the carbon dioxide we can't use the oxygen.

This paradoxical fact is explained in a physiological law called the Verigo-Bohr effect, which states that when levels of carbon dioxide in the blood are lowered, the chemical bond between oxygen and hemoglobin increases. Because hemoglobin won't let go of its oxygen, this makes it hard for the cells of the brain, heart, and kidneys to get the oxygen they need. The consequence is that the deeper you breathe, the less oxygen your body cells will get. We know the results of this kind of overbreathing as hyperventilation. One of Dr. Buteyko's most fascinating discoveries was that all asthmatics overbreathe and that the rate of this overbreathing increases during asthma attacks.

HYPERVENTILATION—THE MISSING LINK

Most of us know from experience what happens when we breathe too much—perhaps when we are blowing up balloons or blowing on the fire—we feel dizzy, we may have palpitations, and if we keep at it, we may get chest pains and even lose consciousness. This is hyperventilation, another name for overbreathing, and it was first described in 1870 by a Dr. Jacob DaCosta who called it the "soldiers' heart syndrome," because he noticed how it caused "disabling shortness of breath and an irritable heart" in soldiers during the American Civil War.

Modern medical and scientific texts have many conflicting definitions of hyperventilation, but from a Buteyko point of view, the key to understanding the term lies in the word itself. *Hyper* means "too much," while *ventilation* refers to "lung ventilation." If you measure the ventilation of your lungs, compare it to the established norm, and if you find that you are breathing above the norm (usually four to six liters of air per minute), then you are hyperventilating.

Medical misunderstanding of hyperventilation is related to the extraordinary fact that most asthma specialists don't know what the norm of lung ventilation should be. This means that the doctors who treat breathing disorders don't know what it is to have truly healthy breathing. They argue that not knowing doesn't matter and that you should "leave it to your body" to establish the breathing norm. Yet if you went to a diabetes specialist and asked what your blood-sugar level should be, he or she would never say, "It doesn't matter; leave it to your body. Oh, and take this and this medicine three times a day. . . ."

Some doctors also argue that rather than hyperventilation causing asthma attacks, asthma attacks induce hyperventilation as the body's natural reaction to lack of oxygen. However, the first trial to measure lung ventilation in the Western world (which took place at the Mater Hospital, Australia, from 1994 to 1995—see Appendix 3, page 162) proved that all asthmatics hyperventilate even when they are not having asthma attacks. To the considerable surprise of many scientists, all thirty-nine asthmatics in the trial had an average intake of fifteen liters of air per minute, three times the norm.

What's more, that same trial demonstrated that patients who learned the unique breath control methods of the

Breath Connection decreased their hyperventilation from fifteen liters per minute to nine liters per minute. As a result of that decrease they were able to reduce their usage of bronchodilator drugs comfortably by 90 percent and of steroid drugs by 50 percent. The control group, which did not use the Breath Connection and did not decrease lung ventilation showed no improvement.

Unfortunately modern medicine recognizes only acute, visible hyperventilation, usually caused by anxiety, but these cases represent a mere 5 percent of hyperventilators. The other 95 percent of people who hyperventilate—encompassing a broad range of slowly developing and cumulative symptoms— are left without treatment.

We have seen how efficient control of our bodies' metabolism depends on maintaining a delicate balance between oxygen and carbon dioxide in our bloodstreams. When we breathe at the appropriate depth and rate—more during exercise, less when we are relaxing—this balance is undisturbed. But when we overbreathe, our levels of carbon dioxide drop dramatically.

Most of us think of the need for oxygen as the key to our breathing, but in fact the level of carbon dioxide is the marker that determines the rate at which we should breathe. The paradox is that while you are taking in more oxygen by overbreathing, that oxygen isn't getting to where it is needed in your body and brain. This is because lack of carbon dioxide causes constriction of the blood vessels, reducing blood supply to the brain and to the rest of the body.

When carbon dioxide levels in the blood go down, so does the acid content of the blood, causing a phenomenon known as "alkaline blood." When the acid/alkali balance of your blood is upset, the results can include bronchospasm, suppression of the immune system in general and the development of allergic reactions in particular, overproduction of mucus, disturbance of the nervous system, loss of oxygenation, and imbalance of the metabolic processes in the bronchial cells, or, in other words, asthma.

So, to sum up, when you hyperventilate, not only does less blood get to important areas of your body, but the oxygen carried by the blood is less easily released there and the low levels of carbon dioxide in the body lead directly to asthma symptoms.

DEEP BREATHING TEST

You may want to try this test yourself, although beware: It may provoke an asthma attack or, if you are epileptic, a fit.

- Sit down and start to breathe fast and deeply through your mouth, as you do when you are running.
- Within thirty to forty seconds (far less for some people) you will develop unpleasant symptoms which may include dizziness, palpitations, rising blood pressure, coughing, and wheezing. (Don't keep this up for long: If you were to keep going you could develop a serious headache, migraine, asthma attack, or you could black out.)
- When you develop these initial symptoms, stop breathing deeply, close your mouth and try to breathe gently through your nose. Your symptoms will go away.
- If you try the test again, you will develop the symptoms again.

The point of this test is that these symptoms are caused not by too much oxygen but by too little carbon dioxide.

In 1909 Professor Yandell Henderson conducted an experiment on a number of perfectly healthy dogs. He put them on breathing machines, which forced them to hyperventilate. They soon started to tremble, as asthmatics do after a dose of nebulizer, and within four to six hours, in spite of having plenty of air, all of them were dead.

In 1952, Dr. Buteyko discovered that hyperventilation is a major cause of asthma. He argued that it is not merely a trigger factor because all asthmatics hyperventilate, whether their asthma is classified as emotional, mild, severe, stress-related, occupational, or triggered by an infection.

Dr. Buteyko also found that all asthmatics recover from asthma when they stop hyperventilating, because when you normalize your breathing you also eliminate bronchospasm, inflammation, and mucus from the lungs. The next time you have an asthma attack—or symptoms such as wheezing or tightness in the chest—take a look at your breathing. You will find that it is much deeper than usual.

TYPES OF BREATHING

- It is a common mistake to divide breathing into diaphragmatic, chest, and stomach breathing, as physiotherapists tend to do.
- We all breath diaphragmatically because the diaphragm is the main breathing muscle which follows commands from our breathing center.
- Breathing from the diaphragm is not going to make you healthier, unless you are advised to breath less, not more.
- There are only two types of breathing: normal and abnormal. The latter leads to disease.

It makes interesting reading to research how close scientists of the past have been to cracking the asthma puzzle—and to making the link between hyperventilation and a range of other diseases. Some scientists have been very near to Dr. Buteyko's discovery that hyperventilation is the cause of many illnesses. Some have tried to understand the powerful effect of carbon dioxide on the body, but there has been too big a gap between their thinking and that of doctors who have traditionally regarded carbon dioxide as a waste gas and who have relied heavily on drugs to treat their patients.

René Laennec (who invented the stethoscope in the first half of the nineteenth century) was closer to the Breath Connection and to the solution of the asthma puzzle than many modern scientists. He concluded that asthma was caused by spasms of the bronchial muscles and that if the asthmatic held his breath, he or she could breathe naturally for one or two breaths after that, clearly demonstrating that the bronchospasm was capable of momentary relaxation. He was very close to understanding that the human body—a very sophisticated chemical factory—is often able to produce the necessary chemicals to heal itself without resorting to the help of drugs.

Today's doctors recognize that by deliberate hyperventilation and overbreathing asthmatics can produce asthma attacks or make their asthma worse. They may put this down to "drying out the airways" or "cooling the airways" (see page 139), while Breath Connection practitioners would say it was lack of carbon dioxide, but what is interesting is that traditional medical practitioners have never tried to prevent asthma by deliberately decreasing hyperventilation.

The articles of Dr. D. Innocenti (in *A Physiotherapist's Textbook*) on chronic hyperventilation syndrome are fifteen years old now, yet many of his observations are not accepted by today's doctors: "Hyperventilation has been recognized for many generations as an acute disorder. . . . Unfortunately, the Chronic Habitual Hyperventilation Syndrome more frequently goes unrecognized. Chronic hyperventilators may be referred to a succession of specialists who find no evidence of organic disease. Many become chronic invalids with gross anxiety neuroses as a result of the continuance of undiagnosed, alarming symptoms. The situation is self-perpetuating in this group of people, who breathe in such a manner that their arterial carbon dioxide level is persistently low; and this may be the basis of a variety of symptoms."

Dr. Innocenti offers this list of some of the symptoms of chronic hyperventilation:

- Cardiovascular symptoms: palpitations, tachycardia, peripheral vasoconstriction
- Respiratory symptoms: bronchospasm, breathlessness, air hunger, excessive sighing, chest pain
- Neurological symptoms: paresthesia, dizziness, lack of coordination, disturbance of vision, disturbance of hearing, blackouts
- Musculoskeletal symptoms: muscle pains, involuntary contractions, tremors, cramps, tetany
- General symptoms: exhaustion, lethargy, weakness, sleep disturbance, headache, disturbance of concentration and memory, anxiety, panic attacks, phobic states, excessive sweating

According to Dr. Buteyko, these are just one tenth of all the symptoms of chronic hyperventilation, which he believes may cause headaches, migraine, chronic fatigue, schizophrenia, and of course, asthma, to name but a few.

There is also a link between hyperventilation and cystic fibrosis—a disease that causes patients to suffer from having very sticky mucus in their lungs. There is a further interesting link between asthma and epilepsy in that hyperventilation is a major cause of attacks or fits for both of these disorders.

According to Anthony Hopkins in his book *Epilepsy,* "one proposed mechanism for the association between stress and seizures is hyperventilation. Matson and colleagues reported three patients who, when anxious, tended to hyperventilate unconsciously. At these times, EEG and clinical seizure activity increased, correlating with a reduction in alveolar $P\,CO_2$. The hypothesis that anxiety leads to hyperventilation and, by lowering $P\,CO_2$, triggers the seizure activity was supported by their observation that administration of 5% carbon dioxide could prevent or terminate the seizure activity, even though anxiety and overbreathing continued."

The fact is that epileptics, like asthmatics and people whose illnesses fall within a range of other related disorders, always hyperventilate. With reconditioning of their breathing patterns through the Buteyko technique, to establish proper levels of carbon dioxide, it is possible to prevent seizures—and asthma attacks—without the use of drugs.

ASTHMA AND HEADACHES

You may have noticed that during an asthma attack, or when you are coughing, or after using bronchodilators, you feel dizzy or develop a headache. This is sometimes considered an insignificant side effect of bronchodilators.

Dr. Buteyko, however, explains that your headache is a result of hyperventilation, to which you are especially prone after a sustained cough or severe asthma attack. What is happening is that lack of carbon dioxide is causing narrowing of the blood vessels in your brain. For the same reason, your heart will be pumping hard, you may be having chest pains, or you may even have a heart attack.

Far from being a side effect of asthma drugs, these are the classic symptoms of hyperventilation.

AN OVERBREATHING SOCIETY

There are a variety of reasons why we develop hyperventilation, or habitual overbreathing, including infections, stress, and medications. But perhaps the most important reason is that we are trained to overbreathe—and we have the habit of overbreathing. Look at the people around you: As they walk down the street nearly all of them breathe through their mouths, an orifice which is bigger than the nose and which takes in far more air. Look at children; their mouths are open, too.

Western culture teaches that deep breathing is good for us. When I ask patients where they got this idea, they say, "It's common knowledge" or "I was brought up to believe this" or "That's what the doctor said." Yet this belief has caused no end of problems. Just as we first dislike alcohol when we first try it but overcome our dislike to develop a taste for it, we also can learn to develop a taste for deep breathing.

If you are taught to breathe deeply, you can override the delicate reflex in your respiratory center, a group of cells located in the medulla of the brain, which is responsible for the regulation of breathing. Your respiratory center then becomes adjusted to a lower level of carbon dioxide, so you learn to feel that this process is normal breathing.

FRESH AIR

Is it good to have all the windows in your house closed in order to have more carbon dioxide? Is it good to be on an overloaded bus where many people are exhaling carbon dioxide? The answer is "no" to both questions because:

- neither of these situations will enable you to increase your level of carbon dioxide. Even if there were ten of you in a telephone booth, the level of carbon dioxide would go up to 0.5 percent, yet if you are asthmatic, you need to raise your level by 2 to 3 percent;
- we need fresh air not because of oxygen (the air around us contains 20 percent oxygen, even on a crowded bus) but because of negative ions. Air conditioners, which also reduce negative ions, are bad for breathing, too;
- people on the crowded bus produce not only carbon dioxide but other gases that are detrimental to breathing.

To take another analogy, many dancers and models have good posture. They need it, so they have cultivated it. The rest of us don't need it, so we don't care about our bad posture. Instead, we visit chiropractors to treat the symptoms of our back pain, and our chiropractors don't mind at all when we come to see them again and again! But visiting a chiropractor will not make your posture better: This is something you have to do for yourself.

It follows that with asthma, medical treatments which address the symptoms will do nothing to change the cause of asthma. There is no medication in existence that can normalize your breathing patterns for you. The Breath Connection, however, can teach you how to normalize your breathing, putting an end to asthma symptoms and the need for medication.

OVERBREATHING AND ASTHMA—A SUMMARY

- Asthma attacks happen when you increase your rate of overbreathing or hyperventilation.
- If you know how to control your hyperventilation, you can overcome an asthma attack.
- If you normalize your breathing you can cure your asthma.
- You can't cure asthma without normalizing your breathing.

LEARNING TO BREATHE AGAIN

Dr. Buteyko teaches that it is possible to relearn correct breathing. Some doctors say that this is impossible because breathing is an involuntary process, and therefore, even if asthmatics do hyperventilate, there is nothing you can do about that.

It is true that many of our bodily mechanisms, including breathing, are controlled by automatic chemical and physical means. But breathing can also respond to our voluntary control. For example, we can hold our breath when swimming underwater, or we can increase our rate of breathing when we blow up balloons.

We all know, too, that there are other nonautomatic factors that can cause us to breathe more, including emotion and stress. Another of these factors is habit.

The Breath Connection teaches us to overcome this habit, to retrain our breathing centers, and to reset our level of breathing to normal levels, with tremendous positive implications for our health in general, and for asthma in particular.

THE ADVANCING EDGE OF RESEARCH

Doctors admit that the present trend of an increasing prevalence of asthma and allergic disorders shows no early signs of reversing, which suggests that those who research the causes of asthma will not lack work for decades to come. Doctors also admit that there is still a good deal of doubt about the mechanisms that cause asthma, especially those concerning the minority of people who do not have allergic asthma.

Still, at intervals, scientists proclaim new departures in asthma research such as the prospect of genetic engineering. Genetic engineering, however, remains many decades away. Meanwhile, the leading edge of research shows that nonallergic asthma patients have a larger number of "helper T lymphocytes" than others. Might it not be possible, speculate asthma researchers, to treat asthma by attacking these helper T cells? Perhaps with new powerful drugs?

What we really should be asking is, What effects are such drugs going to have on hyperventilation? If they decrease hyperventilation, they could be a cure for asthma (providing they do not have major side effects). If they do not decrease hyperventilation, they will eventually cause more harm to asthma sufferers than other, less powerful drugs.

The truth is there is no "magic pill" that can cure asthma, now or in the future. The cause of asthma is hyperventilation, so the best way to prevent it is to retrain your breathing, using the Breath Connection.

3

THE BREATH CONNECTION WORKSHOP

LEARNING THE BREATH CONNECTION

So what is the Breath Connection in practice, and what happens when you or your child participates in a workshop? The science of the Breath Connection is sophisticated, but as the success of the method with small children shows, you don't have to understand the technical details fully to experience a dramatic and rapid improvement in your health. During the workshop, patients learn to recognize their overbreathing patterns and, through breathing exercises, to retrain and recondition their breathing to normal levels. The program includes education about the effects of lifestyle and behavior on breathing, and the causes of hyperventilation are addressed.

The Breath Connection takes discipline, and, yes, it does take time to learn. It is sometimes quite difficult for adults at first, because they have a lifetime of bad breathing habits to overcome, but they soon master it when they realize what excellent results come from a little effort. And the good news is that it is easy for children. Children from the age of four can do it for themselves, and there is a special program that enables parents to help their babies learn normal breathing patterns. Children from the age of five onward get results more quickly than adults, no matter how severe the kids' asthma. It is important that the Breath Connection should be taught only by a certified practitioner, so do ask to see credentials (a diploma or certificate from Dr. Buteyko). The method is taught either in groups or on a one-to-one basis.

WORKSHOP: DAY ONE

During the first session you are asked to fill in various forms so that the practitioner is aware of what asthma medications you are using and of the steroids you have taken or have ceased to take. The practitioner will also want to know about any other illnesses you have, any recent severe asthma attacks, hospital admissions, respiratory arrests, or clinical deaths. (This occurs when a patient is declared biologically dead but is able to be revived by a physician.) Children under the age of sixteen must be accompanied by one or both parents.

Then the Breath Connection practitioner explains the essence of Buteyko's discovery, which is that overbreathing is the cause of asthma. He or she will ask the workshop to try the Deep Breathing Test (see page 37). The test demonstrates that too little carbon dioxide, not too much oxygen, is the cause of the unpleasant symptoms of hyperventilation such as dizziness, coughing, wheezing, and palpitations.

Next, the practitioner explains how to measure your own breathing pattern using the control pause (see box on page 48). The relationship between your control pause, carbon dioxide levels, breathing, and asthma is explained.

THE CONTROL PAUSE—THE MAJOR SYSTEM
FOR MEASURING BREATHING HEALTH

To measure your control pause, sit comfortably in an upright chair, relax and breathe out. Then breathe in normally and out again, holding your nose after the outbreath. Count the seconds, using a stopwatch, until you feel the need to breathe in again. Breathe through your nose without gulping air. The number of seconds you counted before breathing in gives you your control pause.

The ideal control pause is sixty seconds, but a control pause of forty to sixty indicates good health. A control pause of thirty means you are breathing enough for two people and you are mildly asthmatic. A control pause of fifteen indicates that you are breathing for four people: This is serious hyperventilation, with asthma symptoms that are likely to occur every day. A control pause of ten denotes severe asthma with daily and nightly symptoms, medication every day, steroids and hospitalization from time to time, while a control pause of less than five in a person with asthma means you are having an asthma attack—or calling an ambulance!

The practitioner explains that carbon dioxide is a natural bronchodilator or "natural albuterol" (the active ingredient in salbutamol) and also talks about issues such as the Verigo-Bohr effect (see page 34) and the impact of carbon dioxide on the acid-alkali balance of your blood (see page 36).

Then the practitioner explains asthma as one of the results of hyperventilation and describes how your body reacts to the loss of carbon dioxide (which follows overbreathing) by activating a range of defense mechanisms, from mucus production to constriction of the bronchial tubes.

A discussion of asthma medication follows, during which the practitioner makes sure that everybody understands the difference between "relievers" (bronchodilators such as albuterol) and "preventers" (steroids such as prednisone and becotide). It is remarkable how little most people know about their medication, and there is often a great deal of confusion to sort out about the functions of the different drugs and when they should be taken. We advise patients to take relievers only when they need relief, but to take steroids on a regular basis. (For more information about orthodox medication, see Chapter Nine.)

Having covered this important groundwork, the practitioner can now move on to explaining the Buteyko breathing method, which involves a range of exercises to reduce levels of breathing. When the practitioner is sure that everyone understands the basics, the patients practice controlling their breathing for fifteen to twenty minutes.

The exercises can feel strange and difficult to perform, so the practitioner will spend time with each individual, helping everyone in the group to get them right. This skilled personal assessment is crucial to learning the Breath Connection properly, as people may make many individual mistakes as they learn. If these mistakes are not expertly corrected, your breathing may increase even more, making your asthma worse.

At this stage, people in the workshop are clearly very interested in the breathing method but still need answers to many questions about such issues as what effects will weather, allergies, sports, and other factors have on asthma. After answering questions, the practitioner gives "homework"—specific exercises geared to the individual needs of each member of the group, as well as these reminders:

- to be aware of your breathing;
- to use the Breath Connection as natural albuterol (the drug found in the commonly prescribed inhaler Ventolin) in case of any asthma problems, only using your inhaler if a few minutes of Breath Connection breathing methods don't help;
- to breathe through your nose at all times, using tape to keep the mouth closed at night;
- to sleep on your left side with your mouth closed (or for children, on your tummy);
- to stop playing sports for a few days until your asthma improves (see Chapter Eleven);
- to break up your sleep and practice the Breath Connection breathing exercises if you experience asthma attacks at night (see Chapter Five);
- to keep taking steroids and to use an inhaler rather than a nebulizer (see Chapter Nine).

This first session usually lasts for about two hours.

WORKSHOP: DAY TWO

At the beginning of the second day's workshop, the practitioner asks how many of the group successfully used the Breath Connection to prevent or relieve asthma symptoms. Around half the group usually report an improvement: Some managed to head off an asthma attack without using their inhalers, while others had fewer problems than usual, and, having taped their mouths for the night to prevent hyperventilation, enjoyed a good night's sleep for a change!

More than half of the group will usually report that they used less of their reliever drugs. Then the practitioner recaps on the lessons of the day before, going through the control pause and the breathing exercises again to make sure that people are doing these correctly. At this stage, some people are likely to say that they can't keep their mouths closed all the time because their noses are blocked—often because of sinusitis or rhinitis. They are asked to wait: The solution will shortly be revealed!

The practitioner introduces a Breath Connection method of opening the airways as effectively as a few puffs of albuterol. After this exercise, the group finds that wheezing, coughing, and tightness in the chest disappears, while the nose is not blocked up. Another interesting effect is noticeable, too: The group finds that their pulses are going down. This exercise can stop palpitations within a minute and reduce heartbeats from 120 to 80 per minute. The practitioner explains who can do this exercise, when, and for how long, because there are some people who should not do it at all.

Youngsters in the group are taught special children's exercises, which they do with great enthusiasm and enjoyment. Some need to be pushed a little; others need to be slowed down in order to get the greatest benefit from the exercises they are doing.

On this day, as on the next two days, the group practices the newly taught breathing methods a great deal. Again, homework is given, tailored to group members' needs as adults or children and depending on whether their asthma is mild or severe. Some members of the group may be advised to do physical exercise or to play a sport—but to do so without using their inhalers beforehand.

WORKSHOP: DAY THREE

By day three, everyone in the group is feeling much better than they were when they started learning the Breath Connection. Many of them have reduced their need for reliever medicines by 80 to 100 percent. All who have been taping their mouths at night are sleeping better. Many of them (especially those who are overweight) report a reduction or loss of appetite, a consequence of their newly improved metabolic processes.

The practitioner discusses a new approach to food (see Chapter Eight) and explains the basic rule that you should eat only when you feel hungry. He or she gives a brief outline of the foods which are considered "good" and "bad," but avoids spending too much time on this discussion, stressing that breathing is more important than diet.

It is noticeable that children make much faster progress than adults, having spent fewer years being damaged by medication and hyperventilation.

Some patients are keen to stop taking their steroid drugs, but the practitioner works hard to persuade them that they should persevere with steroids—at least until they discuss the matter with their doctor.

Spirits in the group are generally high, as people say they have made it through the day without using reliever drugs for the first time for maybe fifteen or twenty years. Others have been able to play sports—again for the first time—without using their inhalers before and after the exercise.

The practitioner gives out more individually tailored homework. Patients are reminded to visit their doctor after the course to discuss modification of their steroid doses.

WORKSHOP: DAY FOUR

Today, everyone in the group is feeling much better (except perhaps those with emphysema, who are merely feeling better; they will need a little more time before they also feel much better).

Most people have stopped using their reliever medicines, while others have cut their usage by around 90 percent. Some overweight people have lost some weight without making an effort to do so. Everyone's control pause is longer, and hyperventilation has greatly decreased all around. Pulse rates in the group are also down to normal, while people are breathing through their noses without experiencing problems of getting blocked.

Again, we practice the Buteyko breathing exercises, while children may be given some exercises specially designed for their needs, and again the group goes home with individual homework tasks to perform.

WORKSHOP: DAY FIVE

Having checked control pauses and practiced the Breathing Connection, it is time for our farewell talk. There are many questions still to answer such as what other diseases the Breath Connection treats. (The answer is, an enormous number, including high blood pressure, chronic fatigue, epilepsy, and cystic fibrosis.)

Everybody is given a strategy to keep normalizing their breathing, plus advice about what to do about any future problems. The end-of-workshop questionnaire is filled in with many positive comments about being able to give up reliever drugs without fear of asthma—often for the first time in decades.

There are questions, too, about Dr. Buteyko, his life and current circumstances (answered in Chapter One of this book). The group generally wants to talk more about why the Breath Connection is not more widely practiced and why it is still not accepted by the medical profession and asthma "experts." Nearly all of them want to join a Breath Connection support group.

Emotion is high on this last day because the group is so pleased and relieved to have found a way to prevent asthma without drugs. There is much shaking of hands, and sometimes even applause for the practitioner. People who have completed a Breath Connection workshop say that these five days have brought more improvement in alleviating their asthma than a lifetime of medication. This is the Breath Connection.

ESSENTIAL BREATH CONNECTION INFORMATION

- According to the Breath Connection philosophy, asthma is your body's defense mechanism against overbreathing or hyperventilation.
- Modern medicine treats the symptoms of asthma; the Breath Connection treats the cause—which is hyperventilation.
- It doesn't matter how many times you breathe each minute; what matters is how much air you use each minute.
- The way to cure asthma is to normalize your breathing pattern. This means that your Control Pause (see box on page 48) should ideally be sixty seconds when you are at rest.
- To learn the Breath Connection you need to be under the care of a qualified practitioner for a few days.

You can have a hyperventilation problem without developing asthma, but you will have other health problems. The Breath

Connection is also effective for controlling some 150 of the world's most common diseases, which are the diseases from which 90 percent of people suffer.

_____

4

SUCCESS WITH BUTEYKO:
PERSONAL STORIES

So let's hear from some individuals who have tried the Breath Connection, discovered that it can stop asthma in its tracks, and realized that their need for asthma medications has almost (or entirely) disappeared.

Tess Graham, a physiotherapist who lives in Canberra, Australia, has two children with asthma. But after attending a Breath Connection workshop, their symptoms disappeared. Tess has since trained as a certified practitioner and teacher, and she now teaches the Breath Connection full-time.

Tess Graham:

I first read about the Breath Connection in a health magazine. It was all so logical that it immediately made sense to me. As a physiotherapist I had worked with people with asthma for many years, believing they could never get completely better. Physiotherapy traditionally teaches deep breathing and coughing exercises, but I could see that these made asthma worse.

I was very shocked when I found that two out of three of my own children had asthma, even though this problem doesn't run in my family. My daughter Jessie was so ill that she had asthma symptoms daily and was on inhaled steroids and an inhaler (bronchodilator drug). She had been on a nebulizer one week in every three. [We will hear more about these treatments in Chapter Nine.] My son's asthma was worse in the springtime, so at times I had two of them suffering from coughing, wheezing, and asthma attacks, which meant not much sleep for me, either!

But it was Jessie who I felt was really on the edge, and for years I lived in fear for her life. Her asthma could come on quickly, and I wouldn't be more than five minutes away from her at any time. But that was before we discovered the Breath Connection. Our first experience was with individual sessions, and then later we attended a group workshop.

DAY ONE: A RADICAL RETHINK

Jessie was seven years old when I took her to the workshop. There were about ten other wheezy children and a lot of nervous parents, many of whom had been told by their doctors that the Breath Connection wouldn't work. Some were very skeptical and were holding on to their receipts very tightly!

It began with the practitioner, Sasha (Alexander) Stalmatski, introducing the Breath Connection and honoring Dr. Buteyko for his achievements. We went on to discuss the basics of breathing and what he called the "propaganda of deep breathing." He said, "Hands up, those of you who think deep breathing is good for you," and about 90 percent of the people put their hands up.

He went on to explain how deep breathing causes problems. We discussed how even blowing up balloons can make you feel dizzy and how blowing very hard into a peak flow meter can make you cough and make your chest tighten up. We soon got the idea that deep breathing is the root cause of asthma.

From that point the children were put into groups to practice breathing gently and quietly through their noses—having first been taught a breath-holding exercise, which unblocks their noses. Jessie used to be a chronic mouth breather, and there were other kids in the group with goldfish-type mouth postures from years of being openmouthed.

Much of that first session was about reminding the children to shut their mouths. If their noses got blocked, they repeated the unblocking exercise. If their noses weren't blocked, they were opening their mouths from habit.

At the end of that first session, the change was remarkable. The noisy breathing and coughing, the snorting and blowing had stopped. The room was quiet, the mouths were shut. You could have heard a pin drop. I saw this sea of faces, mouths closed. I remember leaving that first session with a sense of unbelievable relief. For years I had felt the fear rise when I heard Jessie start to cough, and now I knew we could get out of this mess. At last I understood what caused her asthma, and I was instantly less fearful for her.

That first night I followed Sasha's instructions to get Jessie to sleep with her mouth shut. We had some exercises to do before bed to make sure that her nose was open, and I put the head of my bed next to hers in an L shape so that I could close her mouth through the night, holding her lips together if necessary and moving her chin.

I kept her lying on her side and made sure she kept her mouth shut. I heard her change from noisy breathing to very quiet nasal breathing. This can be a little bit frightening for mothers at first, because we are so used to listening out for the heavy breathing which reassures us that they are still alive, but I soon learned to love the quietness!

DAY TWO: DELIGHT AND EXCITEMENT

Day two is pretty exciting because parents and children come back to the class, keen to share their experience. They say things like, "He used to grind his teeth and wake up frequently, but last night he didn't" or "My kid had the best sleep in years" or "My kid didn't wake up last night, whereas he usually wakes up about four times." Parents often say their children used to be very restless at night, with a sweaty head and lots of kicking and coughing, but after doing the Buteyko breathing method they sleep so peacefully that they can share a bed with them—without getting kicked all night.

Some parents say their children's bed used to look like a battleground in the morning or that they had nightmares or that they used to wet the bed. Once they learn to sleep with their mouths closed and to breathe gently, all that changes. The parents say, "He played soccer for the first time without his inhaler" or "Mary woke up today and didn't need to blow her nose, whereas she usually needs about ten tissues."

It often happens that, even on day two, parents say, "My child didn't need to use his inhaler for the first time in years." In one recent workshop there was an eleven-year-old boy who had been on a nebulizer two or three times a day since the age of three. Mother and child told me that that day, only day two of the workshop, was the first day in eight years that he hadn't needed that nebulizer. They both had the biggest smiles on their faces.

On day two the exercises can still feel quite awkward, and the practitioner has to remind the kids a lot to shut their mouths. But already they have made progress because on day one, some would have felt suffocated by having to close their mouths. On day two it may still be uncomfortable (in which case they do the nose-unblocking exercises), but often they are opening their mouths because of long habit. It can be difficult, but I've never seen a child get upset during a workshop. I have seen parents in tears however, but those are tears of relief.

DAYS THREE AND FOUR: WORK HARD BUT PLAY, TOO!

These two days follow much the same pattern. We increase the intensity of the exercises, depending on how well the patients are doing and how much they can handle. It is a matter of fine-tuning, which is why you should only learn the Breath Connection's breathing methods with the help of a qualified practitioner.

The group has been doing homework and keeping scores on their exercises. Children come up and say, "Look! This is my best score so far!" They think the scores are great fun because kids tend to be a bit competitive, but I stress that we are all different and they are competing only against themselves.

One of the most exciting things to emerge at about this time is the amazing changes in their pulse rates. Some children come in at the start of the week with pulse rates from 80 beats per minute up to around 130. Adults are often between 80 and 100 beats per minute, which indicates that they are pretty unwell. And we don't take the pulses until group members have been sitting in the workshop for about half an hour, so the pulse rates aren't high because they have rushed to get there.

But by the end of the first session, after half an hour of exercises, most pulses have dropped by at least ten beats, and sometimes twenty, per minute. By the end of the week they are down to a good healthy resting pulse of between sixty and eighty beats per minute. That happens to everybody who practices the Breath Connection because if you normalize your breathing, your whole system becomes more efficient and less stressed, which means that the heart can slow down. This is one of the strongest indicators of the success of the program, and no one can say that it is an imagined, placebo effect.

Another wonderful "side effect" of the Breath Connection is that people who were overweight have often lost weight, because the Breath Connection helps your whole system to regulate itself, making changes in your metabolism and appetite. Alternatively, people who need to put on weight find they have gained a few pounds without trying to do so.

On day three we also learn some variations on the basic breath-holding exercises, and we apply these exercises to practical situations such as being at school (for children) or at work (for adults). Eating, sleeping, being in a smoky room, walking out of a building into cold weather—all these are part of ordinary life, and we discuss what you need to do to keep your breathing under control.

We do role-playing to help children understand what they can do if they are on the soccer field when they need to do their exercises, or in a classroom with a cranky teacher who won't let them practice the Breath Connection. Sometimes the children jog around the room so that we can teach them how to breathe correctly when they are playing sports.

For adults, it may be a matter of pretending they are walking upstairs on the way to work: What happens when you get to the third stair and feel you really have to open your mouth? Even talking a lot—on the phone, or giving a presentation—can increase breathing, so we teach various techniques on how to control it. One of the solutions includes taking your inhaler around with you.

The group dynamic is very important in the workshop because people encourage each other. Sometimes people have slow days or days when they feel tired, but others will say, "I had a slow day yesterday, but today I feel wonderful" or "I felt like that, but then I had a breakthrough." In my group, people come back from earlier workshops to support us— and to show off a little!

DAY FIVE: WHERE DO WE GO FROM HERE?

On day five parents are commenting on the changes among the children. They say, "He looks like a different person." The feeling among the parents is that, having seen the change in their own child, they want everyone to know about the Breath Connection. They have this simple knowledge, and they feel almost like evangelists: They want to spread the word. In our area (Canberra) 80 percent of group members will join the local Breath Connection (Buteyko) Supporters' Association (which now has more members than the local Asthma Foundation group).

On the last day, we also discuss the goals we want to achieve in the future and what to do if asthma symptoms should turn up again. Some people are already 100 percent better; others who may be about 75 percent symptom-free still need to make more progress, and I let them know there will be follow-up sessions and more support available for anyone who needs it.

The progress you make depends on your commitment, the severity of your asthma, and the drugs you have been taking. Asthma, as well as drug therapy, can impair the function of your adrenal system, so your body needs time to repair itself.

There are some very active people who need to do very little after the workshop to maintain their normal breathing, but others need to go on working at it to keep up their best breathing. Some people like to pick a time every day—perhaps when they are watching the evening news on television—to check their breathing and practice their exercises for a few minutes.

Or people may hit a stressful period in their lives, or experience an illness, and they may need to increase the practice of their exercises again for a while. We teach people to monitor their breathing daily and instruct them to continue to carry their medications with them and to use them when necessary.

As for Jessie, at the end of the workshop, she didn't need her inhaler anymore. We were also able to reduce gradually the quantity of steroids she was taking, and she was weaned off them altogether over a period of a few months, with our GP's knowledge. She has been medication-free now for four years, and it has been the most enormous relief!

*Angela, another physiotherapist, attended a workshop in
Scotland as an escort to her elderly mother, who suffered
from asthma:*

My mother has always had a lot of chest complaints, beginning with pneumonia when she was twelve years old. That
left her with weak lungs, and she went on to suffer from
bronchitis. Her asthma started about thirty years ago, but it
was sporadic. She would have a bout and then recover. Then
nine years ago she began taking albuterol on a daily basis.
Her asthma got progressively worse, deteriorating until she
was put on steroid drugs.

Her health was such that she wasn't able to do much exercise. She couldn't do any heavy housework or even walk up
an incline. She couldn't establish a healthy sleeping pattern,
and she was two stone (nearly thirty pounds) overweight.
Gradually, she was becoming disabled. I first heard of the
Breath Connection through a television program, and I
offered to take my mother along to a workshop, every evening
for a week. I went as her escort, on the basis that she is very
shy and not good at going out by herself.

During that first session everything you have ever believed
to be true about breathing is turned on its head. My mother
and other members of the group sat looking a bit stunned
and puzzled at first. But it was remarkable how quickly the
techniques she was taught had an effect on her. It was immediately easier for her to breathe, while within two or three
days she was able to tolerate my cats, who had always caused
her to have an allergic reaction.

After the first evening of the workshop she took salbutamol on one occasion only. She did, however, continue with
her steroid treatment, as recommended by the Buteyko practitioner, for another ten weeks. To get off all asthma drugs

within the space of ten weeks is phenomenal for a lady in her seventies with long-term damage to her lungs.

One of the things that pleased my mother most was that she also lost a stone and a half (twenty-one pounds) within that ten weeks—without making any effort to do so. She found that her appetite just melted away, and she followed instructions not to eat unless she felt hungry. It pleased her, too, that whereas she had always had a very pale, ashen face, she now has little rosy cheeks!

My mother's health is better across the board. She has no more hay fever, her energy levels are higher, her emotional state is better, and she can breathe without asthma symptoms. A lot of the problems that she had put down to her age have disappeared. She went to Blackpool Pier with her partner recently and for the first time in many years she was able to walk up an incline without intense effort and without losing her breath!

Jonathan, aged thirty-two:

I used to have an asthma attack about once a week. I used an inhaler to relieve the symptoms, but I had to be careful in cold weather and after eating certain foods. Asthma runs in my family: My uncle died of an asthma attack.

I have found the Breath Connection to be very good. But you do have to work at it, and if you stop, you feel you need to start doing it again. I practice the breathing exercises twice a day, for ten to fifteen minutes per session.

I've played a lot more sports since doing the Breath Connection, and I'm a lot fitter. I haven't had an asthma attack, and I try to avoid using my inhaler completely. It's nine months since I did the workshop and I've used my inhaler only two or three times since then.

Sharon was ten years old when her mother took her to a workshop:

I was concerned that at the age of ten, Sharon was on albuterol for her wheeziness. In the summer when she also had hay fever, she was on steroids, too; one dose at night, another in the morning. I didn't want my daughter on these drugs, although the doctors assured me the dosage she was on would do her no harm, and yet I knew she needed some form of treatment.

Then we signed up for a Breath Connection workshop, and it was great. I respected the fact that the practitioner told us not to stop her medication; it meant I didn't have to feel threatened or afraid of what they were doing. He stressed that we should keep on with steroids, which are preventers, but that we should only take one puff at a time of reliever medicine [albuterol]. At the same time he explained to us how albuterol made asthma worse by breaking up breathing patterns. He said enough to make me feel that I didn't want my daughter to rely on this drug anymore.

At the first session I was very excited but a bit bewildered. The practitioner gave us the background on Dr. Buteyko in Russia and told us about the trial in Australia, which had such positive results [see Appendix 3, page 162]. He explained that we breathe incorrectly, and then he taught us some breath-holding exercises. We practiced quiet, shallow breathing and learned how to measure our control pause [the major system for measuring breathing health, see box on page 48]. Sharon's control pause was ten seconds at the start of the course, which means she was severely asthmatic, and we put that measure on the computer at home to encourage her. By the end of the week it was forty.

The practitioner also told us to be aware of our breathing,

to close our mouths. He recommended that we tape Sharon's mouth shut at night, and she didn't seem to mind this at all. The feeling of the workshop was so positive; Sharon liked going along.

After a few days the practitioner talked to us about diet and recommended that Sharon avoid milk and fish and eat only when hungry. Sharon was to have no chocolate or milk, and we managed to stick to that.

Every night for half an hour before bedtime she practiced her exercises, then control pause; then she repeated each exercise before taking her pulse. We practiced the exercises every day, twice a day for a minimum of half an hour each time. It takes a bit of discipline to keep it up!

At the moment, some eight months after the course, Sharon has fewer symptoms of asthma and uses less albuterol. She stopped using her inhaler entirely for a while, but this week she has had to start again, so I'm keen to take up the exercises again with her.

Andrew, aged forty:

Although initially a bit skeptical, I have to confirm that after five days I do feel a lot better! The Breath Connection has made me aware of my breathing pattern, and also that I need to relax after my stressful job.

Today I walked three miles without being short of breath or even wheezing. I have stopped taking any medication, whereas I used to be on relievers and preventers. If anything, the Breath Connection has also made me realize that I must not reach for my inhaler at the slightest sign of wheezing.

I am not saying that I am completely cured, but I do definitely feel a lot better than when I started this course. I would recommend this to anyone, whether they are asthmatic or not.

*The Breath Connection, while especially suitable for people
with asthma, can also help with a range of other disorders.
Here, Marjorie Curtis describes how her symptoms of chronic
fatigue disappeared after learning to retrain her breathing:*

I have had Chronic Fatigue Syndrome (CFS) for about eight
years. I've had every conventional and alternative medical
test there is and finally succeeded in getting a diagnosis five
years ago. I've also tried dozens of remedies, both conventional and alternative, but none made any difference.

My symptoms included debilitating fatigue, aching bones
and joints, poor concentration and memory, headaches, feeling too hot or too cold with night sweats, palpitations, and
weight gain. I also had nasal and throat mucus, visual disturbances, dry eyes, nightmares, breathlessness, sweating after
the least physical exertion, and mild sleep apnea. In addition, my thyroid was underactive.

In 1995 I went to a Breath Connection class. I was appalled
by my pathetic results on the first day, which were worse than
some asthmatics in the group (I don't have asthma). But
after just one week I felt better than I had in several years and
my control pause was more than double what it was on my
first day!

I have persisted with the daily exercises, three times a day
for the first three months, and now twice a day. I continue to
achieve longer control pauses. One of the best things about
these exercises is that I am in control, and, if I work hard, I
will get the benefits. The results have been amazing. I am
much fitter now and no longer breathless. I can walk faster
and even run, which I wasn't able to do for many years before
I participated in the workshop. I can also do heavy garden-
ing and housework.

I am sleeping much better now and no longer feel exhausted when I wake up in the mornings. I sleep much less—between five and six hours each night, as I used to before I got CFS—although in the period before I learned the Breath Connection I was sleeping twelve to sixteen hours a night! I certainly no longer have sleep apnea.

I no longer need to sleep in the afternoons and I rarely have nightmares now. My GP has found that I need less thyroxine each day while I have lost more than twenty-two pounds since I did the course. I am less hungry and have lost my craving for sweet things.

The problem of mucus, which used to bother me, is much less, and I can breathe easily at night. My heart palpitations have stopped since I learned the Breath Connection, and I no longer suffer from temperature extremes. I have recently felt well enough to take on professional work again because my mind is very much clearer than it has been in years. I feel really well now.

5

YOU AND YOUR ASTHMA

Now that we have explained the scientific basis of the Breath Connection, we can return to the practical questions of what you can do about your own over-breathing. In this chapter we see why asthma is, in fact, your body's way of defending you against hyperventilation. Between 20 and 30 percent of people have a genetic predisposition to asthma, which makes them react to overbreathing with spasms of the bronchial tubes. If you have asthma, you are one of those people, but you can work with your body (not against it) to prevent this problem on a day-to-day basis.

ASTHMA AS A DEFENSE MECHANISM

Your body has many defense mechanisms to protect it from harm. For instance, if you bang your head against a wall, you feel pain, which tells you to stop: Pain is the message from your body, which stops you from continuing to hurt yourself, and as such, it is not a bad thing.

But suppose you respond to your pain by taking pain-killers. You get a bit of relief at first, but if you keep banging your head against that wall, you will need stronger and ever stronger painkillers. In the long run—because you are treating the symptoms and not the cause—you will end up not only with a serious headache but with side effects from the drugs you have taken. Your "treatment" has not been a success!

This may seem like a silly analogy, but in fact it has many parallels with medical treatments for asthma. Modern asthma drugs treat the symptoms of asthma, but not the cause. Meanwhile, we ignore the message of asthma, which, like pain, is one of our body's natural defense mechanisms— because asthma is essentially your body's way of helping to restrict the amount of air you are breathing.

When you overbreathe—and, as we have seen, you may be breathing at three or four times the healthy rate—the level of carbon dioxide in your body goes down (because you are breathing out too much carbon dioxide). In order to survive, we need to maintain a carbon dioxide level of between 3 and 6.5 percent. If you overbreathe too much for too long, your carbon dioxide level will sink below 3 percent, and you will die. It is asthma that saves you from this fate.

Asthma is the message your body is sending you to stop overbreathing. It makes you wheeze, constricts your bronchial tubes, makes extra mucus, decreases your lung capacity—all in the attempt to stop your breathing out so much carbon dioxide. The symptoms we experienced in the Deep Breathing Test—showing the effects of hyperventilation such as dizziness, blocked nose, palpitations, and so on—are likely to occur, too.

Unfortunately conventional treatments ensure that you override the message of asthma. You are given bronchodilators to open up your airways, and when your body sends you an even stronger message with a stronger asthma attack, you are given stronger bronchodilators to combat the constriction in your chest. These drugs act against your body's own defense mechanism, making it possible for you to exhale even more carbon dioxide, so your asthma gets worse.

Once you understand the meaning of these unquestionably unpleasant symptoms, they can become your friends, because they are giving you some very important information—that you are overbreathing. If you respond to the language of your body by decreasing your breathing to end hyperventilation, the message is not needed anymore, and the symptoms will disappear.

Asthma will go away if you stop overbreathing, just as pain will go away if you stop banging your head against a wall. So listen to that message—and don't shoot the messenger!

DAILY HABITS THAT LESSEN
THE EFFECTS OF ASTHMA

Despite these warnings, you have probably been trying to "beat" your asthma with one or more of the range of prescription asthma drugs. But "beating" your asthma means "beating" your body because asthma is your body's own defense mechanism against overbreathing. So, "If you can't beat them, join them." I suggest that you start by investigating your asthma, to understand how you breathe throughout the day.

Let's start now. Say it is evening while you are reading this page . . .

IN THE EVENING . . .

While you are reading this page,

- **Do keep your mouth closed.** This is especially relevant to some elderly people who have the habit of moving their lips when reading. If you can, hold the book above your face. Dr. Buteyko has observed that looking down increases your breathing (we don't know why, although this could be a reflex), and in addition your eyes will get tired much sooner.

- **Don't lie down** unless you are really sleepy, because lying down will also increase your breathing. (This is because we are naturally upright creatures; just try doing a headstand for a few minutes and you will feel the effects of not being upright on your body!) Stay sitting upright in a chair to read, watch television, think, or meditate. Use your bed only for sleep, and avoid taking sleeping pills. It's best only to go to bed when you feel really sleepy: If insomnia is a problem, the Breath Connection will solve this for you, too.

- **Don't forget to take your steroids** if you had any asthma problems today. You don't yet know the Breath Connection, which will decrease your breathing, so steroids are the best drugs to reduce your breathing artificially in the meantime and to prevent asthma attacks.

- **Don't take a bronchodilator to "prevent" asthma.** This is not a preventive medicine. On the contrary, bronchodilator drugs will expand your bronchial tubes for a few hours, increasing hyperventilation. This means that your body will have to produce phlegm to decrease the resulting loss of carbon dioxide. When, as morning approaches, the bronchodilating effects of the drugs you have taken wear off, you will suffer bronchoconstriction again and produce a lot of phlegm as well.

- **Don't go to bed if your asthma is bad.** Fix it first with steroids to prevent nighttime problems. If you don't do this, asthma will wake you up anyway, as the small asthma problems of the day become major problems during the night.

- **Do make sure your mouth is closed when you go to bed.** As we have seen, breathing through the mouth adds to overbreathing. If necessary, use a micropore surgical tape to keep your mouth shut and to help you determine what is going on while you are asleep. If you wake up in the morning and the tape is still in place, you may not need to tape your mouth again. But if the tape is not there, it means that you opened your mouth in your sleep, and for at least a few hours you have been hyperventilating, losing precious carbon dioxide.

Some people develop a kind of claustrophobia when their mouths are taped, and if you feel anxious about it, tape your mouth for a while before you go to bed—maybe watch television for a bit—so that you can get used to it and feel sure that you are able to breathe through your nose. If it is your child who has asthma, try to explain to your child why you want to put tape across his or her mouth. If your child can't accept the idea, wait until he or she is asleep and then gently shut his mouth and put the tape across it.

Don't worry that your child is going to suffocate because of the tape; if he feels he is not getting enough air, he can take the tape off very easily. Thousands of mothers around the world have tried this method without making any com-

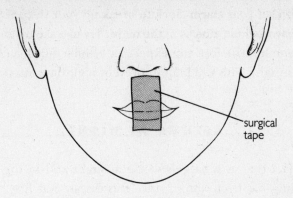

*Taping your mouth helps you check what
is going on while you are asleep*

plaint about it. But if you are still worried, sit beside your child for a while while he sleeps. You will see in the morning that he feels much better after a night in which his mouth was closed, because overbreathing causes far more harm than attempts to normalize it.

- **Do sleep on your left side.** Dr. Buteyko discovered experimentally that this reduces hyperventilation. If your asthma is still bad and you want to sleep, then try to sleep on a chair. This certainly helps, as many severe asthmatics have discovered, because you are in an upright position.
- **Do check your asthmatic child two or three times during the night.** If she has turned over onto her back, turn her onto her side again. If her mouth is open, close it. If her breathing is heavy and wheezy, shake her to "shake off" the hyperventilation and break the pattern of deep breathing.

- **Do set your alarm clock to break up your sleep if you have asthma attacks in the night.** Try to wake up about one hour before you expect an asthma attack and sit upright. This will help to prevent nighttime attacks.

ASTHMA AT NIGHT

The fact that asthma gets worse at night and in the early morning has been known since this disease was first recognized. In the twelfth century Moses Maimonides, who became physician to the Egyptian court, referred to what we would call nocturnal asthma.

The London physician Dr. John Floyer wrote in 1698 about his own attacks of asthma: "I have often observed the fit always to happen after sleep in the night." Floyer's asthma attacks came on exclusively at night, every night, for seven long years!

In the nineteenth century, the distinguished Canadian doctor Sir William Osler wrote that "nocturnal attacks are common. After a few hours of sleep the patient is aroused with a distressing sense of want of breath and a feeling of great oppression in the chest."

Today's doctors describe the phenomenon of wheeziness in the small hours of the morning or on wakening as "the morning dip" and regard this as one of the most characteristic features of asthma. As many as 80 percent of people with asthma are thought to suffer nocturnal symptoms, yet modern medicine doesn't have an explanation for this.

The Breath Connection, however, does offer an explanation for nocturnal asthma. Asthma becomes worse at night and in the early hours of the morning because the horizontal position of your body during sleep increases hyperventilation. Dr. Buteyko believes that this is because the natural position of our bodies is upright. We don't feel "right" while standing on our heads; for related reasons, lying down flat is not the optimum position for our bodies' normal functions.

Contrary to the belief (common among doctors and scientists) that in sleep our breathing is slow and shallow because little oxygen is required, your breathing gets deeper and deeper as you sleep. Watch a sleeping child with asthma, and you will witness this change—or you may even hear it in the form of snoring. Or, set your alarm clock to wake you up during the night, and you will discover that your breathing is deeper than during the day.

The truth is that when we are lying down, our breathing increases, and as a result our levels of carbon dioxide go down. Our bodies respond by trying to retain carbon dioxide, using the defense mechanisms of phlegm and bronchoconstriction. This is why people with asthma often wake up with problems of phlegm, wheezing, tightness in the chest—or with an asthma attack.

Not surprisingly, then, the worst time for asthma is during the wee hours, especially between four and six in the morning, the hours when the death rate from asthma is at its highest.

HELPING YOU GET THROUGH THE NIGHT

Breath Connection practitioners have observed that people with asthma have a better quality of sleep if they sleep on a hard bed (such as a futon) with a thin mattress. Sleeping with a high pile of pillows under your head and shoulders may also help.

Dr. Buteyko also recommends that people with asthma should sleep less and deeply, rather than more and with dreams. How short should your sleep be? The shorter the better. If you can manage on four hours a night, very good. If you can manage on two, so much the better. If you can't face having so little sleep, then just do your best.

- **Don't** go to bed until you are really tired and when you can't do anything except sleep.
- **Don't** go to bed just because it is late. Wait until you really have to sleep.
- **Don't** go to bed during the day. If you have had a sleepless night, which has left you feeling exhausted, just take a nap for twenty or thirty minutes while sitting up in a chair.
- Again, **do** make sure your mouth is closed when you sleep. If necessary, put sticky tape across your lips (see page 74). This may sound strange at first, but try it for one night and you will realize in the morning that this simple method helps to reduce phlegm, helps with snoring problems, provides a refreshing sleep, and helps prevent asthma attacks.

Doctors often argue that you cannot control hyperventilation while you are asleep. But with the Breath Connection, you can certainly control it during your waking hours and with these tips you can also reduce hyperventilation at night. Just as growing children learn how to wake up to go to the toilet rather than wet their beds, so people trained in the Breath Connection develop a kind of guard mechanism that wakes them up when they start breathing too much.

Native American women used to use their fingers to make sure that the mouths of their children were closed when they were asleep, until their children developed the habit of breathing through their noses while sleeping. Doctors of the time noted that these children were often healthier than their colonial contemporaries.

On the other side of the world, the Russian people of four centuries ago slept on short beds with high cushions in the belief that if they lay down flat, their spirit—which in Russian means much the same as "breath"—might leave their bodies.

Dr. Buteyko points out that nearly all animals and birds sleep with their noses or beaks under a paw or wing, knowing instinctively that this is a way to retain more carbon dioxide. Young children who sleep in the "praying position," with their face in their pillows, are doing the same thing, but in Western culture we are unfortunately in the habit of turning children over.

TO SUM UP . . .

- Sleep less.
- Go to bed only when you are really sleepy.
- Never sleep on your back, but on your left-hand side or on your stomach.
- Sleep with your mouth closed, taping it shut if necessary.
- Use the "broken sleep" method when your asthma is bad and/or sleep in a chair.

IN THE MORNING . . .

- **Do get up straight away and try to control your breathing.**
- **Do breathe only through your nose.**

- **Do avoid milk at breakfast time** (and indeed anytime). Use juice on your cereal instead. Dr. Buteyko believes that milk is not necessary to our diet and can be harmful (though a few drops in a cup of coffee won't make much difference if you really feel you can't start the day without it). If you are not hungry, don't eat breakfast. If you are, don't overeat because overeating increases hyperventilation.

- **Do try not to cough.** If possible, suppress your cough or cough very gently with your mouth closed. Coughing is in itself a form of hyperventilation, while hanging on to phlegm is part of your lungs' defense mechanism. Coughing on top of a wheeze will lead to an asthma attack.

- **Do use a bronchodilator if—but only if—you feel tightness in your chest.** You don't yet know the Breath Connection, so use one puff—preferably of Ventolin, because it gives a much lower dose than most other bronchodilators. Only use bronchodilators when you really need them—and as little as possible. If you decrease your dose of bronchodilator, you are taking the first step toward having fewer problems with asthma.

- **Do keep taking your steroids for the time being.** Until you successfully incorporate the methods of the Breath Connection, it is safer to stay on steroids, which artificially decrease your breathing.

- **Do not use your peak flow meter.** This may produce bronchospasm, which shows itself as wheezing or coughing (see page 119).

DURING THE DAY . . .

- **Do keep your mouth closed for breathing**, whether you go out to work or stay at home all day. Remind yourself at intervals; it is important to develop the habit of breathing through your nose to reduce hyperventilation.
- **Do take your steroids now if you forgot them in the morning.** Try never to forget your steroids; far better to forget your bronchodilator—forever.
- **Do breathe through your nose all day long**, whether you are walking, driving, eating, working, resting, or playing a sport.
- **Do check your control pause** (see box on page 48) from time to time, instead of using your peak flow meter. That way you will become familiar with what is happening to your breathing throughout the day, whatever you are doing.
- **Do count how many puffs of bronchodilator you have taken**, and congratulate yourself if you took fewer than usual.

UNDERSTANDING THE PROBLEM IS THE
FIRST STEP TOWARD THE SOLUTION

Even before you start to learn the Breath Connection methods, investigate and get to know your own breathing—and your own asthma:

- Sit down, relax, and start listening to your breathing, in and out.
- How do you *feel* your breath? As a movement of air in your nose? A cooling sensation in your nostrils? Or as a

movement in your chest, abdomen, or head? It doesn't matter how or where you feel your breathing, as long as you can "hear" it and be aware of it.

- Spend as much time as you need to become aware of your breathing: Ten to fifteen minutes will probably be enough.
- Memorize your breathing pattern at rest, when you don't have obvious asthma problems.
- For three days, listen to your asthma in different circumstances:

  in the morning
  during sports
  during lunch
  during an asthma attack or just a wheeze
  during a cough or tightness in the chest
  after using bronchodilators
  before and after using your peak flow meter
  when you have a blocked nose or palpitations or
      a headache
  while you are walking and/or going up stairs
  before and after dinner
  before bed

BE ATTENTIVE AND YOU WILL DISCOVER MANY INTERESTING THINGS

- You will be able to connect different aspects of your breathing with the stages of your asthma.
- You will learn that it is impossible to have an asthma attack unless your breathing is deep.
- You will learn what happens to your breathing when you wake up in the morning because of an asthma attack.

6

ASTHMA AND YOUR NOSE

It has long been known that people with asthma often have nasal problems, too, such as sinusitis, rhinitis, polyps, or adenoids. Modern medicine often treats these associated problems surgically, in the belief that removing the source of chronic infections such as these will restore normal breathing and improve asthma.

Unfortunately many direct nasal treatments, such as the removal of polyps, bring only slight changes to health and it is well known that polyps almost always grow back again after surgery. This is because the root of your problem is still there, not in the sinuses but in hyperventilation.

For polyps, like other nasal problems—and like asthma— are one of your body's defense mechanisms against over-breathing. Learn how to get rid of nasal problems, and you will also learn how to get rid of asthma because these are two facets of the same problem.

What's more, if your doctors do manage to remove your polyps or clear your sinuses, your asthma is likely to get worse, because one of your defenses against overbreathing has also been removed. Indeed, all people with nasal problems and asthma develop their nasal problems before their asthma, while many others go on to develop asthma after having polyps removed.

Look at the progress of this problem step by step, from your body's point of view:

1. You hyperventilate.
2. Your level of carbon dioxide goes down.
3. Your body reacts by causing your nose to become blocked.
4. You unblock your nose using a nasal spray.
5. Your body responds by making polyps in your nose.
6. Your polyps are surgically removed.
7. Your body grows new polyps.
8. The new polyps are surgically removed.
9. Your levels of carbon dioxide are still going down.
10. Your body responds with a new defense mechanism—asthma.

It follows that the more severe your nasal problems are, the more severe your asthma is likely to be, because the bigger your problem of hyperventilation, the stronger your defense mechanisms are going to be, too. The corollary is also true—that some people who have very strong bronchospasms don't have any nasal problems at all—because their bronchospasm is enough of a defense mechanism to make any other unnecessary.

Our bodies' messages come to us like the Four Horsemen of the Apocalypse, and we ignore them at our peril. The First Horseman comes to block your nose, to tell you that you are hyperventilating. But you ignore him, open your mouth, use nasal drops; after all, everyone else breathes through their mouths, and your doctor hasn't told you not to.

So the Second Horseman visits you and gives you mild asthma or polyps—or both. What do you do? Out with the polyps; in with the bronchodilator drugs. Things could be better, but you feel all right.

Then the Third Horseman comes, and he is really angry. His message is a serious one: You have got severe asthma. What do you do? You take your nebulizer, three times a day.

Finally, the fatal Fourth Horseman arrives, and that is the end of your story. . . .

Yet, as we have learned in this book, it doesn't have to be like that. With the Breath Connection, symptoms such as sinusitis and polyps will go away of their own accord, without surgery, when you have learned to recondition your breathing.

After two or three days of practicing the Breath Connection your nasal passages will open up—and stay open. Polyps and sinusitis will disappear within a few weeks. Your doctor may shake his head and say this is impossible. But then he is unlikely to know much about the Breath Connection.

Sinusitis is one of your body's defense mechanisms against hyperventilation. To defend itself against the loss of carbon dioxide, your body constricts the arterial vessels, which carry oxygen-enriched blood through areas such as the brain and the bronchial passages (this may cause you headaches and/or bronchospasm). Meanwhile your body also expands the venous vessels (which carry more carbon dioxide) to areas such as the nose, legs, or anus—which may cause nasal problems, varicose veins, and/or hemorrhoids.

For the same reason—to conserve carbon dioxide—your body grows nasal polyps and develops blocked sinuses, which is why Dr. Buteyko calls sinusitis "asthma in the nose." The symptoms of sinusitis, which include mucus, swelling of the tissues, inability to breathe, even wheezing, are also symptoms suffered by people with asthma.

And just as with asthma, the standard medical treatments for sinusitis address only the symptoms, not the cause. As with asthma the treatments include steroids, as well as "nose dilators" (as opposed to bronchodilators) in the form of nasal drops. But the treatment of nasal problems with chemical sprays only makes the problem worse.

This is because nasal sprays make the tissues (mucous membrane) inside your nose contract, but when the effect of the drug has worn off, your nose responds with a "rebound" effect. In other words, your mucous membrane swells up more than ever before, so you spray more, swell up more, spray more, and so on, in a vicious circle of poor treatment.

HOW TO UNBLOCK YOUR NOSE *WITHOUT* NASAL SPRAYS

This easy method takes only twenty or thirty seconds:
1. Breathe out normally.
2. Hold your breath, close your mouth, and pinch your nose between two fingers.
3. When you can no longer comfortably hold your breath, let go of your nose, but keep your mouth closed and carry on breathing through your nose, which will now be open.

Children and young people can do a dozen or more squats while pinching their noses, or they may walk upstairs while doing this exercise. Adults and elderly people can walk around the house, garden, or office while holding their breath, trying to take as many steps as they can.

Warning: If you start breathing through your mouth after this exercise—in other words, hyperventilating—you may develop wheezing, coughing, or even an asthma attack.

This simple exercise is not part of the Breath Connection technique, but it does demonstrate the miraculous properties of breathing and carbon dioxide.

So what happened during this exercise? When you held your breath, you stopped losing carbon dioxide. The muscular exertion of doing squats or walking helped to increase your raised levels of carbon dioxide still further.

Before the exercise, your nose was blocked by expanded veins (caused by a shortage of carbon dioxide). Raising your levels of carbon dioxide made them return to their healthy, narrowed state, and your nose was unblocked.

This exercise will help your nose to stay unblocked for a few minutes or even hours, but eventually it will become blocked again because, unless you have changed your breathing pattern through the Buteyko technique, you are still hyperventilating and breathing out too much carbon dioxide.

The connection between too little carbon dioxide and a blocked nose is largely unknown to doctors. I once visited a hospital for children with asthma in Sydney, Australia. I met a nice man who was the head of the Respiratory Department there and we had a long discussion about hyperventilation, asthma, and the Breath Connection. He asked me many intelligent questions and agreed with the theoretical part of the Breath Connection's teachings.

But then he said that he could not check how the method worked in his hospital because it entailed breathing through the nose, whereas practically all the children in his care breathed through their mouths—because their noses were blocked.

I told him that I could teach the children how to unblock their noses within a minute. He replied that in all the world's scientific literature there is no reference to the effects of carbon dioxide on a blocked nose. "Sorry," he told me. "I'm very busy. Glad to have met you, and have a nice day."

ASTHMA AND YOUR TONSILS

According to Dr. Buteyko, nearly 90 percent of children with asthma who are six years old or older should have their tonsils surgically removed. Tonsils are supposed to fight infections, which are around us all the time. When an infection reaches the throat the battle begins; tonsils fight the infection, stopping it from getting any farther down into our bodies. In the course of this battle, our tonsils often become large and painful, making it hard for us to swallow. This is a normal response, and it is exactly what we should expect from our tonsils.

So why remove them? Surely we need our tonsils to prevent infections from reaching our lungs? These days it is far from easy to convince ear, nose, and throat specialists that our tonsils—as opposed to our adenoids or polyps—should be removed.

Unfortunately most children with asthma no longer have healthy tonsils that will fight infection. Instead, their tonsils have shrunk. They remain small, and they don't fight infection as they should. Tonsils such as these are not painful, but they are no longer healthy, living tissues. According to Dr. Buteyko, five to six years of hyperventilation (and if your child has asthma you can assume he or she has been hyperventilating for several years already) will "kill" the tonsils. But "dead" tonsils are not harmlessly neutral. On the contrary, they are poisonous to the rest of your body because they exude toxins into the bloodstream, suppressing your immune response. The smaller your tonsils are, the bigger concentration of poison they have. Bad breath—more often attributed to a problem of the digestive system—is actually a sign of dead tonsils, a typical smell of corpses.

Not since biblical times has anyone been able to revive corpses. It is equally impossible to restore dead tonsils to health, so the only way to proceed is to remove them surgically. But beware: Many doctors will try to persuade you to have the adenoids removed at the same time. Don't agree to this: Adenoids are part of your defense mechanism and by practicing the Breath Connection exercises, problems with adenoids will disappear. After a tonsillectomy, people often lose their sickly skin tone and regain a healthy color. The tendency to come down with colds and flu diminishes. You will also find that, after the removal of tonsils, breathing becomes shallower, too.

7

ASTHMA AND ALLERGIES

An allergy is an adverse reaction of the immune system to a substance that most people find harmless. Allergies can manifest themselves in a number of ways, from headache, sneezing, and watery eyes to stuffed sinuses or fatigue—and obviously they can trigger an asthma attack. So why should your immune system be different from, say, your husband's? Why do you cough and sneeze from the smell of cut grass in your backyard, when your husband actually does the mowing and he doesn't react to it at all? The answer lies in understanding that having a strong immune system also means having a normal acid-alkali balance (otherwise known as pH level) in the body. You can break this delicate balance so easily if you overbreathe. You exhale too much carbon dioxide, and, because carbon dioxide is acidic, your body's interior environment becomes too alkaline. Normal *immune* reactions become *allergic* reactions. Hyperventilation can shift your acid/alkali balance within one or two minutes, but by using the principles of the Breath Connection you can restore it to its normal balance.

Allergy is not the *cause* of asthma (see page 22), but it is certainly one of the major *triggers* that may bring on asthma symptoms. Dust mites, cats, dogs, horses, red wine, white bread, gasoline, perfume, cut grass, cigarette smoke, pollution—the list of potential allergens that can trigger asthma goes on and on.

But why is it that some people will suffer from asthma symptoms when they come into contact with these allergens, whereas others can drink, smoke, eat whatever they want, and enjoy life free of symptoms? To deal with allergy we have to understand why this unusual sensitivity is possessed by some people and not others.

The usual medical advice given to people with allergies is to avoid the allergens that induce their allergic symptoms. Sometimes this can be simple: If you know that red wine makes you feel ill, you can drink white wine instead. But often things are not so straightforward. It's not always possible to avoid all the allergens that affect you, and even if you do, other allergens may appear. *For avoiding allergens does not eliminate the cause of allergy.* It reminds me of the story of the boy who was allergic to so many things that he had to live in a protective suit and wear a helmet as if he were an astronaut, and breathe artificial air. He was protected from his trigger factors, but he still had his allergy!

THE BUTEYKO VIEW OF ALLERGY

Dr. Buteyko addresses the problem of allergy from a different perspective. He explains allergy as an imbalance of your immune system and of the metabolic processes of your body. This is caused by a lack of carbon dioxide, which, as we have seen, is a result of hyperventilation. The dust mites or animals that trigger your asthma symptoms are not the *cause* of allergy. It is your immune system's inability to protect you from these and millions of other potential trigger factors in everyday life which is at the root of the problem.

Hyperventilation causes the reactions of your immune system to become abnormal—in other words, you react allergically. But the opposite is also true: As long as your immune system is strong enough, you will not have any allergic reactions—whatever you come into contact with, from cats to French perfume. The Breath Connection normalizes your immune system when it has been weakened by hyperventilation.

ALLERGY AND HYPOSENSITIZATION

Other than avoidance, modern medicine does have one rather controversial method of treating allergy. This method, called "hyposensitization," is in a sense the opposite of the avoidance strategy. It involves injecting you with microdoses of the allergen that affects you, in the hope that this will "educate" your immune system to produce the antibodies needed to fight this foreign substance. This treatment can go on for many years, but it may have few, if any, positive results. This is because your immune system is suppressed by hyperventilation, and hyposensitization is not going to boost your immune system, so it remains unable to deal with allergens.

Moreover, because allergic people are usually allergic to quite a few things, even if you get rid of the reaction to one allergen, you are liable to develop a new allergic reaction to something else—even, perhaps, to your hyposensitization treatment.

Doctors know, or are supposed to know, the danger of this

treatment. Paula Brisco, author of *Asthma: Questions You Have, Answers You Need* (1997), writes: "Desensitization is dangerous because it involves deliberately injecting a substance to which the patient is known to be severely allergic. This can promote severe and dangerous reactions. Formerly there were regular deaths from this procedure and for a time it was completely abandoned in Britain."

Yet some doctors have resumed this treatment, believing it can reduce the amount of drugs a patient needs. Lists of the delayed reactions (which can occur within four to twenty-four hours after the injection) include headache, fever, lethargy, or some wheezing. Should you experience these delayed reactions—or a lengthy reaction—you are advised to contact your doctor or go to a hospital emergency room immediately.

The severe reactions as described by Brisco that can follow desensitization treatment are:

> . . . *chest tightness and a full-blown asthma attack, exceptional difficulty in breathing, hives, stomach pains, difficulty in swallowing, fainting, and nausea. An adrenaline injection, antihistamines, and theophylline may be needed to stop a systemic reaction from progressing to anaphylaxis, or anaphylactic shock, a severe and sometimes fatal systemic reaction.*
>
> *Although deaths from allergy to injections are rare, most of them involve anaphylaxis and lack of resuscitation equipment in the doctor's surgery. For that reason, allergy injections should be administered only in a doctor's surgery where facilities and trained personnel are available to treat life-threatening reaction.*

Even after all this evidence of severe reactions to hyposensitization, as Brisco writes, "no cure for asthma has yet been found. . . . Some doctors call desensitization an inexact, controversial, and dangerous therapy because they don't know in advance whether someone with asthma will benefit from a lengthy series of injections. But other doctors are enthusiastic about desensitization."

How can it be that some doctors remain enthusiastic? The American doctor K. A. Lasko, in his book *The Great Billion Dollar Medical Swindle,* puts forward this theory:

> *These treatments, these weekly shots, these exposures to the thing you cannot tolerate, cost the patient every week. Sometimes the allergic condition actually gets better. Temporarily . . . Fortunately for the allergist, his patients are rarely, if ever, cured. They must keep coming back year after year, week after week. For a shot, for a fee, for what?*

In the United Kingdom and other countries with a national health service, it may not be the individual patient's money that is being wasted, but this is still an unnecessary and costly treatment. It can go on for as long as five years.

Compare this with a five-day Buteyko treatment program, after which you can reduce the amount of medication needed to control asthma and allergies to a tenth of the former level.

A RUSSIAN TALE

The famous Moscow Circus artist Kuklachev used to work with many cats in a show called "Cat House." Unfortunately he was so allergic to cats that whenever he approached them he started to sneeze and his skin became itchy. Because cats were important to his way of making a living and because his job took him all around the world, he tried a wide range of remedies to get rid of his allergies—to no avail. Doctors from many different countries told him the only thing he could do was to get rid of his cats.

Finally, when he realized that Dr. Buteyko treated more than simply asthma, he asked him for help and received treatment.

Two weeks later, Kuklachev was on television with his cats, who were climbing on his head and shoulders, and yet he showed no signs of allergy. "Look what Dr. Buteyko did for me!" he said. "I have no signs of allergy whatsoever. I have visited doctors in Switzerland, Israel, and in America, only to find the cure for my allergy here in Moscow!"

ASTHMA TRIGGERED BY ALLERGY— FIRST LINE OF DEFENSE

It is well known that certain foods, smell, drinks, and so forth can trigger an asthma attack, and a number of people have been rushed to the emergency room or have even died after eating dried apricots, nuts, or chocolate; drinking red wine or a fizzy drink; smelling cats, horses, or cut grass—or interacting with many other things. (Hay fever, by the way, was first "discovered"—described—by a sixteenth-century doctor who noticed that he sneezed and cried after smelling fresh roses.) So what do you do if, say, you have accidentally eaten something which you know will lead to an asthma attack in a few minutes? Alternative treatments cannot give immediate relief in this instance: You need help now, this minute, and should use a conventional medicine such as an antihistamine.

Or, practice the Breath Connection:

- Sit down.
- Breath out.
- Hold your breath for five seconds (count slowly, 1-2-3-4-5).
- Inhale through your nose as gently as you can.
- Exhale through your nose, and hold your breath for ten seconds (again count slowly).
- Inhale gently through your nose.
- Exhale for a count of fifteen.
- Inhale through your nose, and start breathing as shallowly as you can for five minutes. This should increase your carbon dioxide levels, which will restore your acid-based equilibrium, which will stop the allergic reaction, which will stop the asthma attack, which will make you happy!

If this exercise does not bring relief within five minutes, take the medication that has helped you in the past, and plan to take a Breath Connection workshop with a practitioner who can help you use these techniques effectively.

To give one example, I was once having dinner in a Turkish restaurant with a lady who suffered from many allergies and was exceptionally careful in choosing her food—no bread, no red wine, no spinach, no yeast. She could eat almost nothing. But her rice must have been dusted with some flour or additive, and the moment she tried it she developed a reaction. Her breathing got very deep, her chest began to move up and down as if had just been running, and she became breathless and very scared.

I told her to put her hand on her chest and suppress her breathing. She tried but panicked and felt that she couldn't do it. I told her to try not to move her hand. I encouraged her to hold her breath while counting to three silently, then to breathe in and out, for the count of five.

We repeated the exercise together for about twenty minutes. When she was able to breath out for a total count of forty, she felt fine! Normally she would have taken eight to ten puffs on her inhaler to stop the allergic reaction to what she had eaten.

She signed up for a Breath Connection workshop the very next day! And it was a good thing, too. Even I can't teach the Breath Connection method in twenty minutes, and nobody can learn it that fast!

8

ASTHMA AND DIET

Your diet can be an important factor when it comes to asthma—especially the considerations of *when* you eat, and the *way* you eat. There are also some types of food that can make your asthma much worse.

However, when thinking about your diet, do remember that asthma is essentially a breathing disorder, not an eating disorder. Breathing is more immediately vital to us: You can survive for weeks without food but only for a few minutes without breathing. Buteyko practitioners never discuss issues of food or diet with their patients until they are two or three days into a Buteyko course so that the patients have a chance to experience significant improvement in their asthma from learning how to reduce hyperventilation.

THE BREATH CONNECTION DIET

There is one very simple and natural rule at the heart of the Buteyko philosophy about food, and that is, *Eat when you are hungry—and only when you are hungry.* If you are not hungry, do not eat. The reason for this is that if you eat when you are not hungry, your hyperventilation will increase, making your asthma symptoms worse. There is only one situation in which you really *must* eat, and that is if you have hypoglycemia and your blood-sugar level drops.

We have all been told at times, "You must eat your breakfast" or "You must eat to get energy." But forget these exhortations because they do you no good. Your body will tell you when you need to eat: not your husband or your wife, your father or your mother, not a dietitian or a diet book, but your own body.

We are even told, "You must eat because you are sick." Yet no animal will touch food when it is sick. Some people say that they eat breakfast because they are told that they must take their medication in the morning "after eating food." But if you are not hungry, it is better to take your medicine and then drink a glass of water or juice or have a cup of tea.

In the same mistaken tradition, parents often say to their children, "You must eat if you want to grow big," but what they really mean is, "You must eat because I feel better when you eat." Parents sometimes say to me, "My son doesn't eat at all, and if I didn't push him to eat, he wouldn't eat anything." Or they say, "She's never hungry," but children learn to hate eating if they are always pushed to eat. Some parents run the risk of making themselves feel better—but their children feel worse—by making their children eat!

No one can survive without food, and when children are really hungry they will eat. Offer them healthy food—no junk food—and wait until they are ready to eat it. If you push them to eat, you will suppress their natural appetite and disturb their delicate metabolic processes.

Don't eat "up front" if you are not hungry. Having breakfast before you go to work or making your child eat before going out is not a good idea. It is better to give your child a banana or a sandwich to eat later in the day, or to take a snack with you to the office. People say, "If I don't eat breakfast I will be hungry later," but a day is a long time, and you don't know how you are going to feel later.

Simply eat at any time when you are hungry. This means that your body is ready for food, and it will digest food much more easily when you are hungry than when you are not. If you wake up in the middle of the night because you are hungry, get up and have something to eat. Forget the rules about breakfast, lunch, and dinner: Forget about calories. *The issue here is not that overeating gives you too many calories, but that overeating makes you hyperventilate.*

Think back to when you last ate a big lunch or dinner. Didn't you feel breathless afterward? And bear in mind that if you are not hungry, any eating is overeating. So put aside that diet sheet you were given by your dietician or naturopath. You may not *want* to eat as much as they have outlined for you at breakfast or at lunchtime. So don't.

Bear in mind too that while the Breath Connection is essentially a technique for retraining your breathing, many people automatically lose weight when they stop hyperventilating, because for the first time in many years their metabolism has begun to function normally.

So eat as often as you want to, but only when you are . . . what? Yes, *hungry*!

"GOOD" FOODS AND "BAD" FOODS

There are some kinds of food which, according to Dr. Buteyko's observations, can increase your hyperventilation.

These include the high-protein foods such as eggs, cheese, cottage cheese, and, worst of all, fish.

Food and drinks which contain caffeine, such as chocolate, cocoa, tea, coffee, and colas, should also be avoided because they increase hyperventilation, although the odd cup of tea or coffee won't hurt. If you are worried about giving up milk because of the risks of osteoporosis or because you believe your child should be getting plenty of calcium, there are numerous other sources of this mineral. Of course, if you are allergic to any kind of food, avoid it, until you have been trained in the Breath Connection.

According to Dr. Buteyko the foods that should form the basis of your diet are the usual green vegetables, other fresh vegetables (but not too many potatoes), and whole grains such as brown rice. Dr. Buteyko also advocates that we eat more spices such as black pepper, mustard, and sea salt—as well as more onions and garlic.

Salt is good for you if it is sea salt and useless, or even harmful, if it is "table salt." This is because sea salt contains many microelements and minerals. Dr. Buteyko recommends that you should use sea salt for cooking and as a natural remedy for palpitations, coughs, and headaches. Just put a teaspoon of sea salt in a glass of hot water, stir, and drink. You should feel relief from your symptoms within ten or fifteen minutes.

In the West we have been encouraged to eat plenty of fruit, but Dr. Buteyko recommends that you don't overdo it. Some fruits, such as oranges and strawberries, can cause allergic reactions in some people. If some fruits are a problem for you, get your vitamins from vegetables instead.

Dr. Buteyko also believes we should drink as much (or as little) water as we want, depending on whether we are thirsty or not. If you are thirsty, drink until your thirst is satisfied. If you are not thirsty, don't drink at all. Current notions that it is good for us to drink some eight glasses of water a day are not proven. As with food, it is better to listen to your body, which will tell you how much you need to drink.

Dr. Buteyko also says that the best drinking water is made from melted ice, for complex reasons having to do with the crystalline structure of water. Make ice in your own freezer, then let it melt. Drink it, and you will notice the difference for yourself!

BUTEYKO'S RULES FOR EATING

- Eat only when you are hungry.
- Do not overeat.
- Avoid high-protein foods.
- Avoid caffeine (chocolate, coffee, strong tea).
- Avoid milk—any milk, including goat's milk or soy milk, because of the high-protein content.
- Eat plenty of fresh green vegetables and whole grains.
- Use natural sea salt, not table salt.
- Drink water when you are thirsty—and only when you are thirsty.
- *The only "good" food is the food you eat when you are hungry.*

9

THE BUTEYKO VIEW
OF TRADITIONAL MEDICINE
AND THERAPIES: GETTING THE
BEST OUT OF DRUG TREATMENTS

*I firmly believe that if the whole materia medica, as
now used, could be sunk to the bottom of the sea, it
would be all the better for mankind—and all the
worse for the fishes.*
OLIVER WENDELL HOLMES, M.D., 1860

If you take prescription drugs for asthma, like it or not,
you are part of a huge and complex system of doctors,
hospitals, health-service providers, and drug manufac-
turers. This system has many political and economic facets—
from the growth of drug companies to the increase in the
number of asthma institutes—and it is expanding every year.

Yet all drugs—and especially the drugs that many asthmatics take every day—create adverse reactions, some of them

severe. In the United States, eminent doctors have argued that billions of wasted dollars, hundreds of thousands of unnecessary hospitalizations due to harmful side effects of drugs, as well as thousands of unnecessary deaths are the price that society now pays for the promotional excesses of the drug industry.

So let's have a look at the contrast between orthodox treatment and the Breath Connection over the years, and then see what the current asthma drugs can do for you—and how you can feel better with less of them, not more.

THE HISTORY OF ASTHMA AND MODERN MEDICINE

- Fifteenth to the seventeenth century: Asthma regarded as a "slight ailment which promotes longevity." Remedies of the time include horse riding and syrup of garlic.
- Nineteenth century: Henry Salter, the prominent Victorian physician, writes that "asthma never kills." Remedies include tobacco smoking, coffee, gold, morphine, and cold baths.
- 1900–1920: Asthma still not regarded as a fatal disease in many medical schools and institutes.
- 1930s: Epinephrine (a bronchodilator) widely used as a drug treatment for asthma. First deaths from this disease are reported.
- 1940s: Isoproterenol (another bronchodilator) is introduced. Deaths from asthma increase.
- 1948: There is a suggestion that use of epinephrine spray treatment has resulted in a fivefold increase in asthma mortality.

- 1950–1965: Deaths from aminophyllin occur in hospitals in the United Kingdom and the United States.
- 1960s: High-dose isoproterenol is introduced, to be taken through nebulizers. Asthma deaths in New Zealand, Australia, and the United Kingdom follow.
- 1970s: Sale of bronchodilators decreases. Death rate from asthma also decreases.
- 1976: Fenoteral (a long-lasting bronchodilator) introduced in New Zealand. Seven thousand people die per year, over a five-year period.
- 1982: Scientists recognize that home nebulizers can be dangerous, at times fatal.
- 1989: Studies report that inhaled fenoteral is associated with asthma deaths in New Zealand.
- 1993: Cases of sudden respiratory arrest reported in otherwise healthy young asthmatics treated with salmeterol.
- 1994: Inhaled steroids are associated with psychiatric and endocrine disorders.
- 1996: High-dose bronchodilators suspected of interfering with anti-inflammatory and anti-asthma effects of inhaled steroids.

  Concerns raised regarding the safety of salmeterol.

  Evidence that regular use of bronchodilators, even as little as two puffs (200 mcg) a day, may contribute to worsening asthma.

  Inhaled steroids are implicated in contributing to glaucoma.

(Details of relevant research papers can be found in the References section on page 169.)

WHY DIDN'T PEOPLE DIE OF ASTHMA 100 YEARS AGO?

There is a great deal of evidence that asthma was not even considered a potentially fatal illness until this century. On the contrary, early medical books express the view that people with asthma—although sometimes suffering terribly from this disease—actually lived longer than people without asthma!

Before 1920, many leading authorities believed that death from asthma was rare, although deaths from other lung diseases (such as emphysema and obstructive pulmonary disease) were sometimes wrongly attributed to asthma—which in its original definition, simply meant "hard to breathe." Asthma mortality rates in young people were stable for a century before the "epidemic" of asthma deaths in the 1960s.

Since then, despite the advances which medical science claims it has made in understanding the underlying pathophysiological mechanisms of asthma, and in spite of "advances" in drug treatments, deaths from asthma in young patients have not declined, and in some areas of the world they have increased.

Asthma mortality rates began to increase with the commercial development of powerful bronchodilators such as epinephrine and ephedrine and reached a peak in the 1960s with the use and overuse of even more powerful bronchodilators and the nebulizer (an electric pump that delivers a much bigger dose of a bronchodilating drug).

According to the Italian professor V. Serafini, "at this time [1992] when mortality from other chronic diseases is on the decline, clinical observations in recent years have demonstrated an increase in the mortality from asthma in several countries."

In more recent years, the overuse of bronchodilators has been followed by the overuse of steroid drugs—which can also be fatal in the long run. Overdosing on steroids does not kill you immediately, but it may suppress or even destroy the production of natural steroids by your adrenal glands.

Then, because you are reluctant to take yet more steroids (perhaps because of their side effects or because of the current prejudice against them), you may develop steroid deficiency. This in turn can lead to a severe asthma attack, hospitalization, and even death.

Surveys have shown that up to 30 percent of people who die from asthma did not consider themselves to be severely asthmatic. It could well be that they are young people, irritated by their lack of breath during sports or sexual activity or when they have a cold or the flu. So they took one puff of their bronchodilator after another, and then another, and then another and another . . . eventually with tragic consequences.

THE HISTORY OF ASTHMA
AND THE BREATH CONNECTION

Research from 1971 to 1996 establishes that

- hyperventilation and low carbon dioxide (hypocapnia) are common in asthmatics;
- low levels of carbon dioxide are the rule in asthma (until respiratory failure sets in);
- carbon dioxide is a bronchodilator and protects against bronchospasm;
- asthma improves with breathing control;
- tests using peak flow meters are known to cause bronchospasm, making test results unreliable, especially for people with a long history of asthma;

- breathing retraining for people with asthma leads to profound improvements in general health and in asthma in particular.

BRONCHODILATORS

It is some seventy years since physicians started to prescribe the powerful bronchodilator drugs adrenaline and ephedrine to "open the airways" of people with asthma. In that time, different and even more powerful bronchodilators have been developed.

Bronchodilators are also known as "relievers" because they "rescue" you from the unpleasant symptoms of asthma—as opposed to "preventers," the steroid medicines that prevent asthma symptoms. None of these drugs can cure asthma; they can only provide temporary relief from the symptoms.

The best way to keep asthma under control, as most doctors aim to do, is to use a bronchodilator (albuterol is frequently the active ingredient in bronchodilators) for emergencies and to use steroids for prevention of emergencies. It is important that bronchodilators not be used according to a rigid timetable, but only when you feel that you need it, in the same way as you would take a headache tablet for a headache. In other words, if you don't have any asthma symptoms, don't use this drug.

People often give the following reasons for taking bronchodilators:

- I have a low peak flow.
- I need to open up my airways before taking a preventer such as becotide.
- I want to play sports.

- I always take it.
- My doctor recommended it.

But these are not good reasons for taking bronchodilators. Nor is albuterol of any use for a wheeze or cough. It is intended to relieve bronchospasm, not coughing.

Some people who have been taking albuterol for years ask me whether they should cut their dosage in half—or even give it up altogether. My answer is, Just don't take bronchodilators when you don't need them, that's all. Take them when you need them, and take only one puff each time. Why take two puffs as a matter of routine, when it may be absolutely unnecessary to take a double dose?

SHORT-TERM RELIEF, LONG-TERM TROUBLE

It is important to avoid taking bronchodilator drugs unnecessarily for some very good reasons.

- First, they don't cure asthma because they don't address the cause of asthma.
- Second, they can cause nausea, vomiting, loss of appetite, abdominal discomfort, hyperactivity (especially in children), personality changes, rapid pulse, heart irregularity, dizziness, anxiety, delirium, hallucinations, and more.
- Third, and most important, they cause further hyperventilation.
- And fourth, an overdose of bronchodilators can be fatal. Approximately five thousand people now die from asthma every year, and fears have grown in recent years that inappropriate use of bronchodilator drugs

have contributed to the rise in the death rate. In the 1960s, a virtual epidemic of asthma deaths hit Britain. There were (and are) strong suggestions that certain bronchodilators—and large doses of all bronchodilators—led to the epidemic.

Since increasing proportions of asthma-related deaths have been certified by coroners, sudden and unexpected deaths appear to be becoming more frequent, and we must suspect that modern treatment, which is so helpful to most patients, may be a serious hazard to a few. The period of rising mortality coincides with increasing use of both corticosteroid drugs and pressurized bronchodilator aerosols, especially of isoproterenol.

In the 1980s a series of deaths occurred in New Zealand after the introduction of another high-dose bronchodilator. Again, the drug was withdrawn, and the number of deaths dropped. Some years later a study from Canada found that asthma patients using twice the recommended daily dose of bronchodilators had double the risk of a fatal or near-fatal asthma attack. This is thought to be because these drugs can cause increased sensitivity to allergens in what is called the "rebound" effect, as well as long-term deterioration of lung function.

But perhaps the most relevant, but little known, reason for avoiding unnecessary doses of bronchodilators is that although they provide short-term relief, in the long term they make asthma worse. This is because by opening up your airways they make you hyperventilate even more than before, worsening your breathing pattern and causing you more severe problems with asthma in the future.

LONG-TERM RELIEVERS—SERIOUS TROUBLE?

There are worries too about the safety and effectiveness of the new class of bronchodilator, salmeterol. This drug is a long-acting, slow-release bronchodilator that can be taken once every twelve hours and is prescribed only for use on a regular basis, two puffs at a time.

You are supposed to use this drug in the morning and before bed at night, without even knowing whether you are going to need it. Yet this is a powerful drug, at least ten times stronger than albuterol. Surely it is unwise to use it blindly in this way?

Some asthmatics say to me, "But when I use salmeterol I don't need to use albuterol because I don't have any asthma symptoms!" I say, "Well, if you used morphine for a headache, you'd find that it works better than other headache tablets. But there is a problem. Morphine will destroy you—especially if you take it twice a day, every day! And what can help you after morphine? Not an ordinary headache tablet for sure."

IN A NUTSHELL

- Use bronchodilators strictly on a "when required" basis.
- Use the minimum dose to get relief from symptoms.
- Don't use long-lasting bronchodilators.
- If two to three puffs of albuterol don't help you, then take oral steroids.

EMERGENCY ACTION

So what should you do if you are a severe asthmatic and you are having an asthma attack that is so serious that one, two, or even three puffs of albuterol don't help? In such a case you must take oral steroids to prevent further, more serious symptoms, because excessive use of an inhaler is a sign that an even more severe asthma attack is coming on.

STEROIDS

The group of drugs known as steroids (or corticosteroids) was developed earlier this century from the hormone cortisol, which is naturally produced in our bodies by the outer layer of the adrenal gland. The first steroid drug, cortisone, was in fact a natural hormone, and modern corticosteroid drugs are all chemically similar to natural hormones.

Interest in steroids intensified during the 1940s, when researchers found that they could have dramatic results in the treatment of rheumatoid arthritis, and the scientists who had isolated and purified cortisone were awarded the Nobel Prize for Medicine in 1950.

Soon cortisone was being tried for a wide variety of medical conditions—with some striking successes. One of these conditions was asthma. It quickly became clear that steroids could combat severe, life-threatening attacks of asthma. However, disappointing relapses occurred when steroids were withdrawn, and before long it emerged that long-term maintenance treatment was essential in some patients.

But like most powerful drugs, steroids proved to have some major side effects. The most serious of these was that steroids suppress the immune system, making the patient more vulnerable to a host of other diseases. As a result, in the late 1960s there was a reaction against the use of steroids. Nevertheless, these drugs have saved the lives of hundreds of thousands of asthmatics. One intravenous injection of steroids at the hospital during a severe asthma attack makes it possible for you to breathe again—and to survive.

Some people with severe asthma, who have suffered side effects from steroids in the past, now refuse to take these drugs. Yet it is an overdose of steroids that produces side effects. Surviving on the razor's edge of severe asthma, it is only a matter of time before such a person is admitted to a hospital, where, in order to save his or her life, the patient will be given a massive dose of steroids, which in turn will suppress and damage the adrenal glands' production of the patient's own natural steroids. If asthmatics, through fear of side effects, neglect to take more steroids, they may develop steroid deficiency. This in turn may lead to such a severe asthmatic attack that even nebulizers don't help, and so it's back to the hospital again. Sometimes, too late.

In this vicious circle of steroid depletion, hyperventilation is also damaging the adrenal glands. Some asthmatics develop steroid deficiency as a result of serious or prolonged hyperventilation. If they do, they must take artificial steroids or put their lives at risk, just as diabetics must inject insulin when their own natural insulin fails. According to Dr. Buteyko, oral steroids are in fact the best medication for asthma, because steroids are the only drugs which can reduce hyperventilation, addressing the cause of asthma—in contrast to bronchodilators, which increase asthma symptoms.

Dr. Buteyko believes that asthmatics die not from asthma but from hyperventilation caused by two factors:

- Overdose of bronchodilators
- Lack of steroids

SIDE EFFECTS OF STEROIDS

Steroids used in an inhaler have few significant side effects as the dose is very small. However, you may experience:

- hoarseness (the most common complaint)
- candida or "thrush" (a yeastlike fungus in the mouth)
- suppression of growth for some children

Inhaled steroids are now also implicated in the development of psychiatric and endocrine disorders.

Oral steroids can have more serious side effects, including:

- suppression of the body's production of natural steroids
- reactivation of latent infections (such as tuberculosis)
- the breakdown of partly healed stomach or adrenal ulcers
- excessive hairiness (hirsutism)
- a moonlike face
- excessive appetite and weight gain

In addition, if you already have diabetes, osteoporosis, glaucoma, or cataracts, steroids can make any of these diseases worse.

But note that most of these side effects occur as a result of *improper use* of steroids. Taking steroids twice a day, every day for months on end—whether the drugs are needed or not—as many doctors recommend, is the real cause of unpleasant side effects, especially the suppression of your own natural steroids.

HOW STEROIDS WORK

The medical profession admits to understanding little about how steroids work. Unfortunately this lack of understanding has serious implications for the drug treatment of people with asthma because steroids are often given in overdose (too large a quantity) or in underdose (too little).

Fortunately Dr. Buteyko discovered how steroids work. He realized that these drugs decrease breathing, which treats any inflammation, reduces mucus, and helps to relieve bronchospasms.

Steroids are also known to protect against allergy. The Breath Connection teaches that this is because reduction in breathing creates more carbon dioxide in the body, which in turn makes the immune system strong, thus protecting against allergy.

HOW TO MAKE THE MOST OF STEROIDS

The right way to take steroids, according to the Breath Connection, is to take them in response to your condition. As all asthmatics know, their condition can vary a great deal from day to day. Every person with asthma should have a clear understanding of what steroids do, how to take them, and when.

No doctor can monitor your condition on a day-to-day basis, which means it is up to you to assess your own condition and administer the correct dose, according to your condition, your breathing, your control pause, and your pulse. But when your body needs steroids, give it steroids. You need to learn about your own asthma, and to understand the signs that tell you that your body needs steroids—oral or inhaled—now!

This is preferable to developing a "steroid debt" that your body will not forget or forgive. Pay the debt sooner rather than later; if you don't, other people in the hospital will soon pay it for you—and with a massively bigger dose than the one you have been avoiding. The ideal treatment for asthma is to practice the Breath Connection's breathing control and meanwhile to use steroids when necessary. Ultimately the Breath Connection will reduce overbreathing—and therefore inflammation and allergy will also be reduced—while increasing your natural production of steroids. In time, there will be no need to use the artificial steroids any longer.

The wrong way to take steroids is to follow a doctor's schedule or "five-day plan," in which you are told in advance how many steroids to take and when. How does your doctor know what dose you are going to need in three days' time or more? The same goes for inhaled steroids. Some days you will need more than two puffs, twice a day; on other days you will need less.

And why are you being told to take these preventer drugs in the morning, when the night—the most difficult and dangerous time for asthmatics—has already passed? The best time to take steroids is two or three hours before bedtime to prevent early morning problems. (If you have an asthma attack in the morning, however, and find that two or three puffs of Ventolin don't help, take steroids straight away to prevent more serious problems.)

The best way to take oral steroids is to chew up the tablet and wash it down with a drink of warm water (not milk, which is bad for asthma). This helps you to absorb the tablets better with a minimum of irritation to the stomach. You'll feel the effects sooner, too—after two or three hours instead of six or eight. It is usually recommended that you take steroids after eating food, but I have found it is better to take them on an empty stomach.

If you are on a "scheme" that is supposed to reduce your dose of steroids, but you feel that your asthma is getting worse, don't reduce your dose. Increase it instead, and return to that previous level of dosage when you feel better.

Many people with asthma believe they are hooked on steroids and will have to take them for the rest of their lives. This is not true. The good news is that by practicing the Breath Connection so that you achieve a control pause of forty, even people who have been taking big doses of oral steroids are able to get off the steroid hook.

IN A NUTSHELL

To make the best use of steroids
- estimate your condition and establish the correct dosage for you;
- change the dosage daily depending on how you improve or deteriorate.

Explain this plan to your doctor, who should help you to follow it.

CROMOLYN DRUGS

When the first commercial cromolyn drug appeared in the 1960s, it was hailed as a revolution in asthma treatment: "Asthma cure discovered!" proclaimed the newspaper headlines. Alas, nothing so remarkable has happened, and the great revolution has failed.

Cromolyn, which doctors believe has little if any effect on adults, is commonly prescribed for children with asthma. Doctors argue that cromolyn has few significant side effects and often recommend it as a preferred line of treatment before steroids.

Yet very little is known about how this drug works, and according to Dr. Buteyko, it does have significant side effects. He found that it makes the bronchial tubes inflexible, comparable to the lung damage suffered by people who have worked in the mining or cement industries. He also found that these drugs may cause bronchitis after just a few weeks of regular use.

To sum up, these drugs don't stop asthma attacks and they don't reduce breathing (as steroids do). Don't use them.

METHYLXANTHINES

This group of drugs, which includes the asthma medications theophylline and aminophylline, can also open up your airways. Theophylline, like caffeine, stimulates your central nervous system. How bronchodilators work is not fully understood, but it is known that theophylline relaxes bronchial muscles when given in the correct dosage.

Unfortunately, too much theophylline can cause convulsions and, ultimately, death. Children and old people are most vulnerable to the severe side effects of an overdose of theophylline because of the complexity of selecting the correct dose. When used in conjunction with inhaled bronchodilators, as some doctors recommend, these drugs can be fatal.

Under the circumstances, the most important thing I can say about these drugs is don't use them.

PEAK FLOW METERS

A peak flow meter is a device used—either at home or in your doctor's office—to measure the volume of your "forced expiration." In other words, you blow into it as hard as you can to produce a reading, which tells you your ability to blow out air. A lot of air is considered "good."

But not only can peak flow meters be harmful to people with asthma; the devices' results are also unreliable and misleading, telling you nothing about your breathing patterns or about hyperventilation. They can also set up a vicious circle of needing more bronchodilators to maintain a good peak flow, therefore increasing hyperventilation and, in turn, asthma symptoms. One study (Gayrard et al., see References, page 169) described peak flow as "a crude measure of bronchoconstriction," which "cannot alone provide conclusive evidence of asthma."

Many people with asthma develop wheezing, coughing, and/or tightness in the chest after using a peak flow meter. This is because when you blow into the device, you blow out a lot of carbon dioxide, which switches on your body's defense mechanism of bronchoconstriction.

Many people have great peak flow figures—when they feel well or when they have just used a nebulizer—but they may be struck by an asthma attack within hours. In fact, the bigger your lung capacity, the bigger your potential for hyperventilation—hence, the worse your asthma attack may be. Developing a good lung capacity can certainly help you in sports or running or carrying a piano up to the sixth floor, but it's better to get rid of your asthma first. (It's worth noting, too, that some nonasthmatics have a small peak flow.)

Doctors underline the necessity to maintain good peak flow figures, but if you enter this never-ending battle you are bound to lose. Say your peak flow reading is 400 (which is considered pretty good for asthmatics). To maintain this figure, you take asthma drugs such as bronchodilators, which increase your hyperventilation and make your asthma symptoms worse in the long run. The logic of this situation is that you have to keep increasing your dose of asthma drugs—which means increasing your asthma problem—in order to keep up your peak flow readings. Clearly, a no-win scenario.

Alternatively you can measure your asthma by checking your control pause (see box on page 48). Your control pause is far more relevant to your problem—and safer, too.

PHYSIOTHERAPY

Many people who end up in hospital after an asthma attack are offered physiotherapy as a form of treatment for their symptoms. Alternatively some doctors will refer their asthmatic patients to physiotherapists for in-office treatment. Although there has been very little research to demonstrate the effectiveness of physiotherapy in the treatment of asthma, it has been used for decades.

Unfortunately physiotherapy for asthma involves teaching you to breathe more deeply—in the belief that you need more oxygen. It also involves "coughing therapy," in which the physiotherapist teaches you how to cough in order to remove mucus from your lungs.

However, not only do both these techniques increase hyperventilation, making asthma worse, but, by removing mucus, physiotherapy is also working against one of your body's defense mechanisms against loss of carbon dioxide.

In Australia, at the time of writing this new edition, around a dozen physiotherapists have stopped treating asthmatics with these techniques and have instead turned to the Breath Connection (see case study on page 56).

My advice on physiotherapy for asthma: Don't use it.

COMPLEMENTARY TREATMENTS

This book is not the place to discuss these treatments in detail, but from a Buteyko point of view the main principle to consider is what effect do complementary therapies have on breathing?

Any therapy that increases breathing, such as physiotherapy, rebirthing (which involves deep breathing), blowing up balloons—as practiced in some hospitals—is harmful. Any breathing exercises that should be called deep-breathing exercises are harmful. If you have asthma, you don't need any practice at deep breathing; you've already been doing it for years!

Any therapy that decreases breathing even indirectly and temporarily—such as relaxation, meditation, the Alexander technique, acupuncture, massage, a vegetarian diet (because eating protein increases hyperventilation), fasting (because eating increases hyperventilation), Tai Chi (which is relaxing)—will do you good rather than bad.

Yoga is a wonderful way to control body, mind, and spirit and can therefore be very beneficial for people with asthma. Most yoga positions and exercises help you to retain carbon dioxide because the positions you are required to hold reduce breathing. Unfortunately most Western yoga teachers recommend deep or "full" breathing, which they believe will help you get more oxygen.

A true yogi, by contrast, should be able to control breathing, with the capacity to breathe very deeply, very shallowly, or hardly at all. But these are exercises for special effects. What counts is the breathing of a yogi when he is not doing these yoga exercises. What is his breathing pattern? It should be very shallow and superficial.

Wonderful as yoga can be, there is one problem: As a therapy it is too empirical. In other words, you don't know where you are going or what is going on with your breathing. Like other forms of relaxation and meditation, it is good for lowering your breathing for an hour or more each day, but you breathe for twenty-four hours a day. What really counts is what is happening to your breathing during the other twenty-three.

Some therapies, such as traditional Chinese medicine, homeopathy, and yoga, can be good or bad, depending upon the practitioner. Exercise can be good or bad, depending on whether you have learned to control your breathing using Breath Connection techniques.

Other self-help methods of reducing asthma are simple and effective common sense:

- Get rid of any chronic infection you may have.
- Get rid of carpets that attract dust and other allergens.
- Breathe through your nose.
- Avoid stress.
- Eat healthy food, not mass-produced junk.

A CURE FOR ASTHMA?

From the beginning of recorded history, people have tried to combat the symptoms of asthma with all sorts of weird and wonderful potions. Some of the first ever "asthma medications" contained chemical compounds that have been reproduced in modern drugs: Others seem totally grotesque and bizarre to us today. But what will history's verdict be on the massive doses of bronchodilators and steroids handed out with full confidence by twentieth-century doctors? Will they seem any less strange? Time will tell.

- Four thousand years ago, the Chinese doctor Ma Huan was making medicines for asthma from the herb ephedra. The asthma drug ephedrine—derived from the same plant— was rediscovered in Japan in 1914 and is still in use.

- The influential physician Galen, born in Asia Minor in 131 A.D., recommended owl's blood in wine as the best remedy for asthma.

- Sir John Floyer, the prominent British physician, included a list of asthma remedies in his *Treatise of the Asthma* (1698), such as "Gil and Hyslop," "Syrop of Sulphor," and "Spirit of Harshorn"—as well as bleeding and purging. His treatise was translated into French and German and had a great influence on English clinicians of the eighteenth century.

- Other eighteenth-century remedies for asthma included "Syrop of Garlick," "Tincture of Lavender," "Smoked Amber with Tobacco," and "Gentle Vomiting."

- By the nineteenth century, people with asthma were being dosed with a wide range of potions from chloroform and belladonna to strong coffee, tobacco, and alcohol.

- In 1863 the physician Henry Salter wrote about "the treatment of the asthmatic paroxysm by full doses of alcohol." He described the case of an asthmatic woman who seemed to be beyond all help. He had tried everything—chloroform, ipecac, strong coffee, iodide of potassium, tobacco smoked in a pipe, cigars—but nothing worked. Only when she was recommended to try gin did she apparently gain instant relief from her symptoms!

- In 1834 the *Edinburgh Medical Journal* came close to understanding what we now know to be triggers for asthma when they gave "scientific" reasons for why people with asthma should not use feather pillows. The journal reported an "urgent case of asthma [which] appeared to be induced by electricity excited by new feathers."

- Victorian doctors used bloodletting, cold baths, mineral water, electricity, and magnetism to treat asthma—all in vain.

- Chloroform became a very fashionable remedy after Queen Victoria inhaled it during the birth of Prince Leopold. Indeed, *Anesthesia* was a popular girls' name for years to come. But in 1833 an encyclopedia of practical medicine had warned doctors that chloroform was a "remedy not free from risk." It wasn't until 1928, however, that the august *British Medical Journal* confirmed that view by reporting a few deaths of asthmatics from using chloroform.

- Toward the end of the nineteenth century, a Dr. Oliver discovered epinephrine. Sir Henry Dale purified the chemical messenger it contains, and epinephrine—together with ephedrine—were used as powerful bronchodilators from the 1920s onward.

- In North America, a number of folk remedies were available for asthma, as reported in *Magical Medicine* (1907) by W. Hand:

    Nebraskans kept cats to "catch" their asthma.

    Texans blew into the mouths of frogs before daylight, believing that the frog would die of their asthma, leaving them cured.

    New Yorkers nailed a lock of the asthmatic's hair to a tree in the hope that the tree would die but that the asthmatic would be well.

Nova Scotians stood in the hot blood of a slaughtered animal to cure asthma.

The early inhabitants of Los Angeles thought that owning Chihuahua dogs was the solution.

In Kentucky and Oregon, people measured their children against the wall in the hope—familiar to modern parents and doctors—that when children grew, they would "outgrow" their asthma.

- In 1997, thousands of Indian people lined up for a folk cure for asthma, which involved swallowing a live goldfish, which in turn was supposed to "swallow" the asthma as it went down.

Yet through all these centuries and with all these misconceived ideas, most people did not die of asthma.

GOING TO THE HOSPITAL

What happens when you arrive at the hospital, with a severe asthma attack? Naturally you expect the best available treatment and care. But whether or not you will get it is another matter. Let's run through the typical treatment.

The first step in the management of your acute condition will probably be to give you a bronchodilator drug, administered either by a nebulizer or by injection. If you show any signs of oxygen deficiency or an unusually fast pulse, you will most likely be given oxygen through a mask. Almost everyone admitted to a hospital for an asthma attack is given oxygen in this way. But few doctors understand why you have an oxygen shortfall in the first place. During a severe asthma attack, you are suffering from a lack of oxygen because you are hyperventilating acutely. Artificial administration of oxygen makes you feel even worse, so your condition gets worse, not better, and you may develop bronchospasm.

More dangerous still is the fact that oxygen therapy can cause pulmonary collapse and respiratory failure. This is because when a high concentration of oxygen is breathed for many hours, it is toxic to the tiny air sacs (alveoli) and blood vessels (pulmonary capillaries) in the lungs. Another effect of administering pure oxygen is to cause nausea, ringing in the ears, and twitching of the face, symptoms that warn of convulsions to come. The fact that pure oxygen is toxic has been known for a hundred years, yet it is still being used.

You will still not have received a steroid drug, and this delay, I believe, is one of the main causes of death from asthma. Only after all other measures have failed—after about an hour of ineffective, even damaging treatments—are steroids used.

Even if you have been given steroids and your condition has improved, a nurse is likely to come around every hour to put you on a nebulizer, giving you a large dose of bronchodilators to make you hyperventilate again. Then a physiotherapist may be called in to "help you with coughing." But this so-called coughing technique is yet another way to make you hyperventilate more—again causing loss of oxygen and leading to bronchospasm.

HOW TO SURVIVE IN THE HOSPITAL

Dr. Buteyko advises that you insist on the following treatment, should you ever be admitted to the hospital with an asthma attack:

- Make sure you are given an intravenous steroid drug as soon as possible, after they put you on a nebulizer, which is almost unavoidable. You will feel better within a few minutes, after which you will be able to refuse a routine nebulizer treatment.
- Accept treatment with a nebulizer only if you feel you really need it and for just enough time to get relief from your symptoms.
- Refuse to take oxygen.
- Refuse any physiotherapy that involves blowing up balloons, coughing therapy, and other forms of hyper-ventilation.

Of course, it can be very difficult to assert your wishes under the circumstances of an acute asthma attack, so it may be wise to brief your partner or relatives so that they can communicate what you want as well as keep an eye on your continuing treatment. (Remember Dr. Semmelweis?)

AFTER THE HOSPITAL

The two weeks after leaving the hospital are an anxious time, with a high risk of relapsing into acute asthma. Why should this be the case? Again, the misuse and misunderstanding of steroids is the root of the problem.

Usually you are advised that after leaving the hospital you should take a high daily dose of steroids, say 50 mg, and then reduce that dose by 5 mg every three days. Or, you may be prescribed what doctors call a "steroid burst" for five days only, stopping steroids completely after this time. You may also be given a complicated combination of nebulizers and long-acting bronchodilators.

The trouble is, no matter how good your doctor is, he or she cannot know what will happen to you in three days' time after you have been discharged from the hospital. Your asthma may get worse, but according to your doctor's plan, you have to decrease your dose of steroids. It could be that on the very day when you are supposed to stop taking steroids altogether, you feel really terrible because you have got the flu, or a cold, or your asthma got worse.

Logically this is a time at which you should be increasing your steroid dose, but your plan tells you to decrease it—or stop it. So what happens next? The hospital again. This scenario raises serious questions:

- As we are all different, why are we all prescribed the same 50 mg dose of steroids after we leave the hospital?
- Why give us five days to come off steroids—as opposed to three, or seven, or nine—regardless of our condition?

The answer to both of these questions is that doctors don't understand how steroids work, they don't know how to detect steroid deficiency or to prescribe the correct dose, and they don't like steroids.

The sad implications of this lack of knowledge about steroids is that they are not used when really needed—resulting in deaths from asthma—and that when they are used, they are often given in overdose, causing the unpleasant symptoms that made people want to avoid them in the first place.

DEAR DOCTOR

Sooner rather than later you should discuss the philosophy of the Breath Connection with your doctor. The following points, which you could put in the form of a letter, might help you to approach him or her fully armed with the scientific facts. (Should you wish to study the subject further, seek out some of the published papers listed in the References section at the back of this book.)

- Asthma is a breathing disorder.
- According to scientific international norms, I am supposed to breathe between four and six liters of air in one minute while I am at rest. I breathe three times as much as this (as demonstrated by my minute volume).
- I am overbreathing, which means that while I am taking in more oxygen, less oxygen is actually getting to certain areas of my brain and body (Verigo-Bohr effect, see page 34).
- At the same time, I am exhaling too much carbon dioxide, which is a smooth-muscle relaxant and bronchodilator. This means that my bronchial tubes become constricted.
- As a result of the bronchoconstriction I have been prescribed chemical bronchodilators, which have been implicated in recent asthma deaths and rising morbidity.
- In 1952, Dr. Buteyko invented a method to change breathing patterns, which could be a drug-free solution to my overbreathing problem.
- The Breath Connection underwent a scientific trial in Australia, from 1994 to 1995, showing an unprecedented 90 percent reduction in the use of bronchodilators, together with a 50 percent reduction in the use of steroids, by the asthmatics in the trial. The control group, using conventional medicines, showed no reduction in use of bronchodilators or steroids.

- When I start learning the breathing techniques taught in the Breath Connection workshop, I must keep taking my steroid medication, and I should use my "reliever" (bronchodilator) medicine only when I feel that I need it.
- I plan to learn how to use breathing techniques—in which carbon dioxide acts as a natural albuterol—to stop the symptoms of asthma. I will keep my inhaler in my pocket just in case. I will use it if I need to use it, but I hope I never have to again.
- Once I have been free from asthma symptoms for a few weeks, I will ask you to reduce my dose of steroids.

Your doctor may be skeptical—indeed you may be skeptical to start with—but it is quite likely that he or she will say, "This is just a matter of breathing, so why not try it?"

10

ASTHMA AND YOUR CHILD

Earlier in this book we saw how many of the conventional medical approaches to asthma simply don't work because they fail to address the fundamental cause of asthma, which is overbreathing. It follows that conventional medicine will have many "solutions" to your child's asthma that are, in fact, useless—or even harmful.

In this chapter we look at how the Breath Connection can help your child overcome the frightening and upsetting symptoms of asthma, while for the most part steering clear of drugs.

AN INHERITED PROBLEM?

We're all aware that asthma tends to run in families. The evidence points to the fact that there is a genetic predisposition for asthma in people, which may determine whether or not you will have the disease. Fortunately, this is *no more than a predisposition which may or may not result in asthma.*

The conventional medical view is that when people with this asthma gene (or genes) come into contact with an environmental trigger, asthma is the result. The Breath Connection operates on the principle that *hyperventilation is the root cause of breathing problems* in those susceptible people who develop symptoms of asthma.

According to Dr. Buteyko, up to 50 percent of children in families where one parent is asthmatic may develop asthma. The figure goes up to 90 percent in families where both parents are asthmatic. His view is that newborn children do not have asthma, but that they may develop asthma after a few months of hyperventilation.

However, the Breath Connection can stop your child's asthma, whatever his or her genetic inheritance, by tackling the basic problem of overbreathing.

STARTING IN THE WOMB: ASTHMA AND PREGNANCY

If you are a pregnant woman with asthma, you may find that your asthma symptoms improve during pregnancy, or, unfortunately, you may find the reverse. There is no hard and fast rule about how asthma affects pregnant women: Some feel better; some feel worse; others feel no difference at all.

What is clear, however, is that it is possible to prevent asthma problems from developing in your unborn baby by using the Breath Connection techniques. Nature has established a perfect but delicate balance of carbon dioxide and oxygen in the womb, which ensures that the fetus does not become ill. The level of carbon dioxide in the womb is, in fact, twice as high as the postnatal level, while the level of oxygen is five times less than the level after birth.

Hyperventilation in the mother can break this delicate balance, causing—according to Dr. Buteyko—a range of health problems. He argues that if you overbreathe, the oxygen available to the baby decreases, resulting in problems that may be as serious as miscarriage.

While many women find that focusing on their breathing can be of help during labor, it is important to avoid any deep breathing exercises during pregnancy and birth that will increase hyperventilation. Dr. Buteyko's view is that, rather than deep breathing, it is shallow, controlled, nasal breathing that can decrease pain in labor because higher carbon dioxide levels in the blood relax the muscles.

When the baby of a woman who has been habitually hyperventilating emerges into the world, the baby, too, may start life by hyperventilating. She doesn't yet have asthma, but in as little as four months, she may start to show the first signs of this disease.

And as explained elsewhere in this book, the remedies are straightforward. Make sure that her mouth stays closed to reduce hyperventilation, and do not overfeed her. Should she need to take asthma medicines, avoid using a nebulizer on a regular basis: Use it strictly according to need and for as short a time as possible. Better still, use a spacer (a device to help infants inhale asthma medications) rather than a nebulizer.

WHEEZY BRONCHITIS OR ASTHMA?

Many people with bronchitis also have a wheeze, and this combination tends to confuse doctors. What is it? they wonder—asthma or just wheezy bronchitis (bronchitis with mucus that produces a wheezy cough)?

These days—in contrast to treatment forty odd years ago—doctors tend to treat children with wheezy bronchitis as if they have asthma. (In the past, doctors thought the term *asthma* might alarm parents, so they usually avoided using it. In any case, treatment for asthma was in the early stages and not very advanced.)

As a consequence of the confusion surrounding this diagnosis today, children with what was formerly known as wheezy bronchitis are often prescribed asthma drugs. Within a few weeks they become real asthmatics because their medication has made them hyperventilate even more than before.

So what should you do if your child develops a wheeze? Dr. Buteyko recommends that you don't try to get rid of the wheeze artificially with drugs or herbal remedies, or your child will develop asthma as the next available defense mechanism against hyperventilation.

Instead, decrease your child's breathing using the Breath Connection's techniques and the wheeze will disappear by itself.

Be reassured that the wheeze in itself is not dangerous: It is merely the audible signal of your child's body that all is not well. Only in emergencies or when your child is experiencing obvious breathing difficulties should you give your child asthma medication.

Conversely, according to Dr. Buteyko, children with asthma may develop bronchitis as a result of regular inhalation of cromolyn drugs. (See page 117.)

ONCE UPON A TIME:
A SAD CHILDREN'S STORY

The story of what happens to a typical child with asthma, who is treated with conventional medicine, rarely makes for happy reading. It all begins when the child is still in the womb. Because his mother has been overbreathing, her baby develops oxygen deficiency. When he is born, he may be put in an oxygen chamber to "remedy" this problem, but as we have seen (see pages 125–126), this solution only makes the symptoms worse. As pure oxygen is known to "burn" the lungs— even of adults—this baby is already on the road to developing breathing problems in the future.

After birth, too, there are further factors that contribute to overbreathing in babies, such as mouth breathing and overfeeding—not to mention the radically changed environment. The baby has left the safety of the womb's high carbon dioxide for an atmosphere that has far higher levels of oxygen (20 percent) in proportion to carbon dioxide (0.03 percent).

If the baby should develop a wheeze, the doctor may prescribe bronchodilators—to be administered through a nebulizer three times a day, regardless of the baby's condition. This means more hyperventilation for the child and a higher chance of developing asthma.

But life goes on, and the baby becomes a child who can use a cromolyn drug through an inhaler. (Alternatively he may be put on a nebulizer or spacer with a pressurized inhaler.) By the time this little boy goes to school, he should be able to use a drug powder inhaler or autohaler. By now, he may have developed bronchitis as a result of the cromolyn drugs, which are very damaging to the bronchi.

By now our little boy has asthma and bronchitis and takes bronchodilators and steroids regularly, according to a timetable rather than according to need. This is in spite of the fact that bronchodilators increase hyperventilation (the cause of the asthma), and in spite of the fact that too many steroids cause the suppression of the body's own natural steroids.

Meanwhile, everyone from coaches to teachers to physiotherapists—even doctors—is incorrectly teaching the little boy that deep breathing is good for him—instead of teaching him that he should close his mouth, breathe through his nose, and avoid overbreathing.

He may also be taking medicines or herbal remedies to try to get rid of the phlegm caused by his bronchitis. Or he may be simply trying to cough the phlegm up. Either way, he will be making his hyperventilation problem worse. And whether he coughs or takes medicines, the phlegm will still be there again in the morning, trying to protect him from further loss of carbon dioxide.

Now his doctor decides the time for stronger medicines has come, so the little boy is prescribed a long-acting bronchodilator that keeps his bronchial tubes open for twelve hours at a stretch. The result is even greater hyperventilation, even worse asthma, and so the round of nebulizers, hospitals, and massive doses of steroids begins. In the hospital they may put him on the nebulizer every hour (despite the fact the nebulizers have been linked to the deaths of thousands of people in New Zealand during the 1980s). He is also likely to be given oxygen in the hospital, again adding to his asthma problems. In addition, the huge doses of steroids given to him in the hospital have made him moon-faced.

After he leaves the hospital, he is put on a regime of nebulizers and oral steroids. But because the bronchodilator drugs in nebulizers increase hyperventilation while steroids decrease it, this is rather like being given medicine for diarrhea and constipation at the same time. The mechanism which regulates his breathing is now thoroughly confused.

His steroids have been prescribed for five days only, regardless of his individual needs, although he must stay on the bronchodilator drugs. The result is that in a few weeks' time, when the effects of the steroids finally wear off, his condition deteriorates. He has another severe asthma attack. The ambulance is called, and it's back to the hospital again for more oxygen, more nebulizers, more steroids—and so on in a vicious circle of ever-worsening asthma.

For most modern children to date, this has been a story without a happy ending. Now, however, the Breath Connection offers an alternative: a healthy life free of asthma symptoms and free of drugs.

PREVENTING AND ENDING YOUR CHILD'S ASTHMA

In conclusion, there are a number of practical day-to-day steps that you can take to stop your child becoming ill with asthma:

- Teach your child to keep his or her mouth closed, reducing hyperventilation. Ask your child's teacher to remind him or her of the practice while at school.
- Make sure your child remembers to take preventive medicines (steroids) before going to school. Children don't see the immediate benefit of taking these medicines, so they tend to think they're not important.
- Your child should always have an inhaler in her school bag or pocket to use when she can't breathe.
- Teach your child to use reliever medicines (inhalers) only when needed, one puff at a time.

- Your child should not play sports if she needs to use an inhaler first. After completing the Breath Connection workshop, she will be able to play any sport without using reliever medicines first.

- Let the school know that you don't want your child to be put on a nebulizer, except in an extreme situation— for instance, when he is still in difficulties after three puffs of reliever medicine. This is, in fact, an emergency, and you should hurry to take your child home, give him steroids, and take him to a good doctor who will not put him on a nebulizer three times a day.

- Children as young as three are capable of taking reliever medicine through an inhaler, which is preferable to a nebulizer, which dispenses much larger doses of bronchodilator medicine. (Fifty times more, in fact: One puff of the average bronchodilator gives 100 mcg, while a dose of nebulizer is 5 mg.) And because delivery is more efficient through a nebulizer, the effects may be even more powerful. But for infants who really need a dose of reliever medicine, just a few seconds on a nebulizer may be necessary.

- Make sure that you explain all you know about asthma to your child. Some children treat inhalers as toys, passing them around the playground to other kids who may or may not have asthma. If they understood more about asthma, perhaps they wouldn't do that.

- Teach your child how to remedy a blocked nose by pinching his nose and holding his breath (see box on page 86).

- Enroll your child in a Breath Connection workshop and practice the exercises together.

11

ASTHMA AND EXERCISE

Modern medicine has a variety of explanations for the phenomenon of what it calls "exercise-induced asthma." As far back as the Roman Empire it was recognized that asthma was related to exercise, while the prominent seventeenth-century British physician Sir John Floyer linked asthma with emotional stress, laughter, and exercise. Today, doctors try to explain this link in terms of "drying out of the airways," which they argue follows the faster, deeper breathing induced by exercise or laughter.

I once attended an asthma conference in Sydney, organized by the Australian Asthma Foundation. The hall was full of health professionals and asthmatics, despite the hefty conference fee. We heard the usual explanations of the virtues of a new drug treatment for asthma, and then someone asked one professor, "Why do I have asthma attacks when I'm physically active?"

The professor said, "Because your breathing during sports cools down your airways."

Then another person asked, "If I were to exercise in a sauna, does that mean I would not develop asthma?"

The professor thought for a minute and then said, "No, you would develop asthma because the temperature there would still be low enough to cool your airways." Quite a few people in the hall nearly developed laughter-induced asthma at that reply.

So why *do* people with asthma have problems when they run or laugh, even when the warm air of a sauna and/or the effects of running in fog or rain are not enough to stop their airways from drying out? The Breath Connection solves this age-old problem.

Dr. Buteyko points out that if you look at the breathing of somebody who runs or laughs or walks upstairs, or plays a sport—or who argues, shouts, feels fearful, or coughs—you will see that the breathing has one common element in all these modes: hyperventilation. Indeed, many children have learned that they can bring on an asthma attack by crying or by some of the other means just mentioned—quite useful as a way to manipulate your parents or avoid going to school!

HOW TO WALK UPHILL—OR UPSTAIRS— WHEN YOU HAVE ASTHMA

Walking uphill, or even upstairs, can be a real problem for people with severe asthma. Your breathing may become very deep, inducing coughing and wheezing. You are left short of breath and in need of your inhaler.

To avoid these problems, we recommend you follow these simple steps:

- Do not use an inhaler beforehand. Use it when you need it.
- Breathe strictly through your nose as you walk uphill and breathe as little as possible.
- Walk slowly at first, listening to your own breathing and stopping to rest whenever you feel that you have lost control of your breath.
- Once you have reached the top of the hill or stairs, try not to take a deep breath but try to hold back your breathing.
- When you can make it to the top in one go without having to stop and rest, then you can try to go faster. As long as you stay in control of your breath, you are safe.

Basically, your ability to walk uphill or upstairs depends upon your control pause. If your control pause is less than five seconds, you will find it hard even to walk across the room. But if it should go as high as fifty, you would probably be able to run up to the fifth floor with your mouth closed—and still have no asthma symptoms.

The question remains whether exercise benefits people with asthma or not. There are other related questions, too, such as, If sports are good for you, what is the best sport to participate in? And what about using your inhaler before playing a sport: Is this a good idea?

Sports can be either beneficial or harmful, depending on the level of carbon dioxide that you are left with after exercising.

THE EFFECT OF EXERCISE
ON YOUR ASTHMA

Let's look at what is going on with your breathing when you take exercise.

- First, your breathing becomes fast and deep. You exhale more carbon dioxide than usual, so your bronchial tubes become narrowed.

  Moderate and severe asthmatics don't generally have enough carbon dioxide to get past this stage, because their carbon dioxide levels are already so low that any further depletion switches on the body's defense mechanisms in the form of asthma symptoms.

  Mild asthmatics may have sufficient reserves of carbon dioxide to go through this stage.

- Second, the activity of your muscles speeds up your metabolic processes so that your body starts producing more carbon dioxide, which in turn opens up your bronchial tubes.

  If you exercise long enough, your level of carbon dioxide may become higher than it was before you started, so you feel great. This effect may last for a few minutes or several hours, depending on your ability to control your breathing.

- Third, after stopping exercise, your breathing is still deep but your muscles have stopped producing carbon dioxide, making this a crucial time for people with asthma. The positive effects of the exercise may stay with you if you can control your breathing, but if you breathe out too much of the carbon dioxide that you accumulated during exercise, you are likely to develop an asthma attack.

To find out how sports affects your asthma, check your carbon dioxide level fifteen to twenty minutes after exercising. The method is the same as at other times: by measuring your control pause (see box on page 48).

Say your control pause was twenty before taking exercise. (I wouldn't advocate that you play a sport if the control pause is any lower because you are likely to have an asthma attack.) Things could go one of two ways. Either your control pause will increase to around twenty-three, twenty-five, or even higher. Or it will go down to around ten (which means you are wheezing and coughing), or as low as five (which means you are having an asthma attack).

IS SWIMMING GOOD FOR PEOPLE WITH ASTHMA?

It is a commonly held view that swimming is an especially good sport for people with asthma, and it's true that there have been Olympic swimming champions who are asthmatics. Many of the Australian swimming team have asthma. They swim for a few hours a day, every day, for years, and yet they still have asthma, and they still take drugs to treat their symptoms.

The optimistic way to look at this is that asthma can't stop you from becoming an Olympic champion. On the other hand, pessimists might think, Even though I can become an Olympic champion, I can't stop my asthma!

So is swimming good for you or not? Apart from the fact that some people develop sensitivity to the chlorine used to sterilize swimming-pool water, swimming can be good for you. That is, if you can control your breathing so that your carbon dioxide levels stay higher after swimming than they were before you started.

But if that is not the case, you are likely to end up with further asthma symptoms. Indeed, some people with asthma have asthma attacks before they have even left the swimming pool.

WHAT IS THE BEST SPORT FOR ASTHMATICS?

So what is the best sport for asthma? There really is no "best" sport, because what counts is not the sport, but your breath control. Some sports are more amenable than others to your efforts to control your breathing, however. Rhythmical exercise such as jogging, running, swimming, aerobics, and cycling enable you to build up carbon dioxide through the activity of your muscles, while giving you the chance to slow down or stop to get your breath back.

By contrast, sports such as football and tennis, which involve sudden, erratic bursts of speed, make it harder for you to control your breathing.

One of the best sports for people with asthma is horseback riding, because the physical bumping of your body against the horse as it trots breaks up your breathing into fast and shallow rhythms, rather than the more dangerous deep breathing of some other sports.

One of the worst activities for asthma is chess! It is useless from the exercise point of view, and it induces hyperventilation.

DOS AND DON'TS OF SPORTS AND ASTHMA

- Don't use your inhaler before playing a sport. If you can't play a sport without using your inhaler, it means your body doesn't like it, recognizes the danger, and makes its protest through asthma. For the time being, it's better not to play a sport at all. Once you have put an end to your asthma—which takes only a few days with the Breath Connection—then you can exercise without using drugs.

- Do breathe through your nose, keeping your mouth closed, whatever sport you undertake. Breathe only through your nose, and if you feel that your need for breath is so great that you have to open your mouth to breathe, slow down or stop. The urge to open your mouth to breathe is a worrying sign: The next stage along this route may be an asthma attack.

- If you go swimming, ignore the standard advice to breathe in through your nose and out through your mouth. Instead, keep your mouth closed for the breast stroke and back stroke, and for the crawl, try to hold your face under water for four, six, or even eight strokes.

- Do try to hold back your breathing after taking exercise. Remember, an asthma attack may happen only when you are breathing deeply. If you can control your breathing, you can control your asthma.

- Do check your control pause before and after playing sports. Then, instead of following the mantra that "sports are good for asthma," you can measure how good each individual sport is for your asthma—or not good, as the case may be. (A particular sport could, of course, have quite a different impact on somebody else.)

THEORETICAL UNDERSTANDING BEHIND THE BREATH CONNECTION

The Breath Connection represents a development of the hyperventilation syndrome theory. This theory is based on the contemporary understanding of the immense biological role of the carbon dioxide gas in the human organism.

The human metabolism developed in the ancient geological eras when carbon dioxide in the air and water was represented in tenths of a percent. It is probably due to this factor that a definite concentration of CO_2 (7% approx.) must be an absolutely essential condition of each human cell in order for it to sustain all the normal pathways of the biochemical processes.

The problem faced by the evolving human organism has been the depletion of CO_2 in our atmosphere from the tenths of a percent of ancient eras to the current level (1982) of

0.03 percent. Human evolution has dealt with this dilemma by creating an autonomous internal air environment within the alveolar spaces of the lungs. These alveoli contain around 6.5 percent of CO_2, quite a contrast to the surrounding air. The gaseous mix in the womb is also an interesting indicator of the ideal human environment. Here there exists between 7 and 8 percent of CO_2. Dr. Buteyko was asked to speak on this subject at the World Congress of Biochemistry that took place in Moscow in 1972.

CURRENT PHYSIOLOGICAL UNDERSTANDING

1. CO_2 is, through the conversion into carbonic acid, the most important buffer system in the body's regulation of its acid-base balance (acid-alkali balance). A low level of CO_2 may lead to alkalosis. If the level of CO_2 lowers to below 3 percent, shifting the pH to 8, then the whole organism dies.

2. A low level of CO_2 causes a displacement of the oxyhemoglobin dissociation curve, thereby not allowing correct oxygenation of the tissues and vital organs (Verigo-Bohr effect).

3. Poor oxygenation leads to hypoxia and a whole gamut of medical disorders.

4. CO_2 is a smooth-muscle vessel dilator. Therefore a shortfall of CO_2 causes spasming of brain tissue, bronchus tissue, etc.

5. Hyperventilation causes a progressive loss of CO_2. The higher the breathing, the lower the CO_2 level.

6. CO_2 is the catalyst to the body's metabolic processes, playing a vital role in biosynthesis of amino acids

and their amides, lipids, carbohydrates, etc. This is explained in more detail in "The Biochemical Basis of K. P. Buteyko's Theory of the Disease of Deep Respiration."

Through an understanding of current physiology we should begin to see the links between CO_2 and oxygenation of the body, CO_2 and disease. It is clear that a deepening of the breathing does not mean an increase in oxygen uptake. On the contrary, it means a decrease in oxygenation, which leads to hypoxia, imbalance in the acid-alkali balance, and cell spasming.

The fifth point of physiological understanding explains the destructively poisonous influence that hyperventilation has on the organism. It shows us clearly (in conjunction with the other points) that overbreathing leads to imbalance in the body and general deterioration of health.

THE DANGERS OF HYPERVENTILATION

The term *hyperventilation* should be clearly defined. It is not reserved only to the most extreme and visible cases. Hyperventilation simply means "an increase in the function of the lungs above the normal recommended amount." The significance of Buteyko's discoveries hinge on the diagnosis of what Buteyko termed *hidden hyperventilation*, that is, long-term overbreathing that is not clearly visible in the patient.

If a patient hyperventilating 30 lt./min. can receive disastrous physical repercussions in the very short term, then it should be understood that overbreathing 5–10 lt./min. will have equally dire consequences over the long term. The average asthmatic overbreathes between three to five times the recommended amount, sometimes more.

The detrimental influence of deep breathing on the organism is a direct result of the creation of a CO_2 deficit. This has been proven by many experiments, starting with the work of the well-known physiologist Dr. Yandell Henderson in 1909. In his experiments, animals were mechanically induced to breathe deeply and died as a result.

ACID-ALKALI BALANCE

Through its conversion into carbonic add, CO_2 is the most vital player in the maintaining of the body's acid-base balance. Lowering CO_2 in the lungs by deep breathing shifts the body's pH toward alkalinity, which changes the rate of activity of all body ferments and vitamins. An alkaline system is more susceptible to viruses and allergies. The shift in the rate of metabolic regulator activity disturbs the normal flow of metabolic processes and leads to the death of the cell. As mentioned before, if the level of CO_2 is lowered below 3 percent, shifting pH to 8, the whole of the organism dies.

HYPERVENTILATION, DISEASE, AND MODERN MEDICINE

Symptoms of various combined disturbances in the organism of a deep-breathing person are exceptionally diverse. The traditional methods of disease analysis have resulted in the various symptoms of overbreathing—bronchospasms, heart-muscle spasms, increased or decreased arterial pressures, fainting spells with convulsions—being called separate ill-nesses, such as bronchial asthma, angina pectoris, hyperten-sion, allergies, etc. The latter named all lead to complications; for example, sclerosis of the lungs and vessels, myocardial infarcts, and strokes.

The theory of the diseases of deep breathing has previ-ously been presented in a lecture entitled "On Discovery of the Deep Breathing Being the Principal Reason for Allergies, Sclerosis, Psychosis, Tuberculosis, Pre-cancerous Conditions and Other Symptoms of Disease."

In that lecture Dr. Buteyko mentioned that his discovery is not only represented in the method of treatment of the diseases, but in the exposure of their causes. Dr. Buteyko believes that modern medicine has slipped to the levels of blind empiricism. This appears to have happened because attempts to find the causes of diseases such as asthma, angina pectoris, hypertension, etc., have been fruitless; therefore, an important principle of medicine is being trampled on. The very principle upon which the Buteyko philosophy is based: "Having not found the reason of the disease, the physician has no right to treat the patient. Only having dis-covered the reason for the disease is it possible to guarantee the recovery."

Modern medicine, as it stands at the moment, has either stopped looking for the causes of asthma, angina pectoris, hypertension, etc., or it has a false impression of these dis-eases' sources. That is why these diseases continue to remain incurable. Through understanding trigger factors we can only hope to treat the problem symptomatically. Only through the understanding of the cause of the disease can we hope to cure it.

It has eventuated, through Dr. Buteyko's research, that deep breathing is directly linked to at least 150 diseases.

Buteyko has conducted extensive research and has found that diseases such as asthma, hypertension, angina pectoris, myocardial infarcts, strokes, hemorrhoids, eczema, among others, are all symptoms of the imbalance created by deep breathing. In cases where Buteyko's patients had these diseases, they have all been cured, as was proven in the Saint Petersburg and Moscow approbations (see page 154). The Buteyko theory cites that these diseases are the body's defense mechanisms against the excessive loss of CO_2 through overventilation.

THE NERVOUS SYSTEM

The lowering of CO_2 in the nerve cells heightens the threshold of their excitability, alerting all branches of the nervous system and rendering it extraordinarily sensitive to outside stimuli. This leads to irritability, sleeplessness, stress problems, unfounded anxiety fears, allergic reactions, etc. Concurrent with this, the breathing center in the brain is further stimulated, thereby causing a further loss of CO_2. In this way another vicious cycle has commenced.

THE CAUSES OF DEEP BREATHING

Having touched directly on the physiological problems of hyperventilation, and the resulting "blowing off" of CO_2, obvious questions arise: What is the cause of deep breathing itself? What is hyperventilation a consequence of?

There are several factors known to induce deepening of the breath. The most important factor, in Buteyko's opinion, is the propaganda of the usefulness of deep breathing. The contemporary person is taught to breathe deeply even before he is born, when his mother is sent for sessions of deep-breathing exercises during her pregnancy. Often the new-born is encouraged to increase his breathing by having his little arms raised and lowered. And so it follows on, in kindergartens, schools, armies, sports, etc. Deep breathing is encouraged without any scientific basis for doing so.

There are other factors that promote deep breathing as well—overeating, especially of animal protein (fish, chicken, eggs, milk, and, naturally, red meat), sharply increases breathing. It should be noted that food in the form of animal products increase the breathing more than food in the form of plant products; cooked food increases deep breathing more than raw.

Another factor deepening the breath is a state of limited mobility, lack of physical work or activity, idleness. Physical activity encourages the release of CO_2 from the cells, increasing its levels in the body. The breath is deepened by hydrodynamics, by bedrest regimes, by prolonged horizontal positions (especially lying on the back), and prolonged sleep. Recommendations for longer periods of sleep and even sleep therapy have never cured anybody. Most attacks of epilepsy, asthma, myocardial infarction, strokes, paralysis, etc., occur toward the end of sleep, around five A.M.

Further factors deepening the breath are the various emotions either positive or negative, stress, heat, stuffy environments. And the other way around, calmness, temperance, cold temperatures, all assist the shallow breathing.

THE AIM OF THE BREATH CONNECTION

The aim of the Breath Connection is to correct the patient's breathing pattern, that is, recondition the breathing pattern to internationally recommended physiological levels. Through this process the shortfall of CO_2 is also rectified. The process is completely safe and drug-free.

In contrast to the dangers of low CO_2, if the depth of breathing is decreased to below normal and the level of CO_2 in the organism is above normal by 0.5–1.0 percent, there are no negative symptoms manifested. On the contrary, those afflicted with the heavy consequences of deep breathing—bronchial asthma, angina pectoris, hypertension—develop symptoms of superendurance with higher than normal levels of CO_2. The Buteyko and Breath Connection clinics have been regularly observing this for the second decade now. It is evident that decreasing of the depth of breathing does not result in any kind of undesirable occurrences.

What is the normal or correct amount of air we should be breathing? This varies from person to person, although 3–4 liters per minute is the average.

For a more comprehensive analysis of the physiological role of CO_2, please read "The Biochemical Basis of K. P. Buteyko's Theory of the Disease of Deep Respiration."

THE RESULTS OF THE APPROBATION OF THE BBL METHOD IN THE DEPARTMENT OF CHILDREN'S DISEASES IN THE FIRST MOSCOW MEDICAL INSTITUTE OF E. M. SECHENOV

BY K. P. BUTEYKO AND V. A. GENINA

The BBL method was tested and approved by the Medical Institute of E. N. Sechenov between February 27, 1981, and May 21, 1981.

The method is based on a conscious decrease in deep breathing and specifically designed for patients suffering from bronchial asthma. It is based on the fact that clinical results show improvement proportional to the decrease in lung ventilation.

CLINICAL CHARACTERIZATIONS
OF PATIENTS WITH BRONCHIAL ASTHMA

The experiment was based on patients suffering from regular asthma attacks (once a day or more) during the previous month. Some of the patients had severe asthma leading to asphyxia. The purpose of the experiment was to demonstrate the relationship between the major symptoms of the disease (bronchospasm, cough, nasal blockage, and so on) and hyperventilation. The patients were asked to undergo a three-stage hyperventilation test (developed by Dr. Buteyko in 1968).

1. The test was conducted in a sitting position. The patients were asked to use the BBL method. Correctly followed instructions yielded the following results: In one to five minutes there was a decrease or disappearance of the symptoms of asthma; the patients experienced relief from asphyxia, wheezing, cough, or rhinitis.
2. The second stage involved a reverse process; the patients were asked to breathe deeply for fifteen to sixty seconds until the first symptoms of an attack.
3. The patients were asked to repeat the BBL and thus prevent the onset of the attack independently.

If the patients did not understand the relationship between the hyperventilation and the disease, the test was repeated. The test was not conducted if the patients took a bronchodilator 1.5–2 hours prior to the test. Fifty-two patients between the ages of 3 and 15 were treated according to the BBL method: 36 boys (69%) and 16 girls (31%). See Table I.

Of the 52 children, 34 (65%) were hospitalized, 18 (35%) were outpatients. Twenty-four (46%) had atopic bronchial asthma; 22 (42%) had mixed bronchial asthma; and 6 (12%) had bacterial allergy bronchial asthma. The majority of the patients (36) had been suffering from this condition for up to 5 years, 12 for 6–10 years, and 4 for 11–15 years. The patients were divided into three categories: mild, severe, and very severe (see Table II).

Table I—Age and sex distribution of patients

Group	Number	Sex M	(F)	Age 3–5	6–10	11–15
Hospital	34	24	(10)	2	18	14
Ambulatory	18	12	(6)	5	12	1
Total	52	36	(16)	7	30	15

Table II—Patient distribution according to degree of asthma

Group	Number	Mild test	%	Severe test	%	Very severe test	%
Hospital	34	0	0	24	70.6	10	29.4
Ambulatory	18	1	5.5	13	72.2	4	22.0
Total	52	1	1.9	37	71.1	14	26.9

According to patients' histories, 41 cases (79%) had had pneumonia 1–7 times; 4 (8%) were taking corticosteroids (prednisone tablets) prior to the BBL treatment; 6 (11%) were physically handicapped; 9 (17%) were obese; all the children had bad posture. Eleven (21%) had chest deformity; 33 of the children (64%) had allergic reactions to medications; 34 (65%) had allergic reactions to food; and 25 (48%) had allergic reactions to dust. Twenty-seven (52%) suffered from rhinitis; 18 (35%) had Quincke's edema; 47 (90%) had a predisposition to colds and the flu. All had problems with breathing through the nose; 36 (69%) had chronic tonsillitis; 11 (21%) had sinus problems; 23 (44%) had frequent headaches; all had palpitations; and 13 (25%) had unstable body temperature.

Acute periods of their condition were accompanied by the following symptoms: 31 (59%) had sleeping problems; 16 (31%) had loss of appetite; and 13 (25%) had constipation. Of the 52 children, 47 (90%) were regular hospital patients and only 5 (10%) did not require hospitalization.

Prior to the BBL treatment, all children had antibiotic treatment; all had to use bronchodilators; 37 (71.2%) were using [a cromolyn drug] over prolonged periods; 15 (29%) were taking antihistamines. All these treatments were having little effect.

The course of the BBL treatment consisted of a daily training of forty to ninety minutes exercise in the mornings, under the supervision of the specialist; self-training included three to five hours under the supervision of the instructor or the parents. The majority of the children mastered the method in five to ten minutes: They were eager, disciplined, and enthusiastic.

After one to five days of the BBL treatment, the patients were able to stop their asthma attacks, coughs, blocked noses, and wheezing. The patients were encouraged to use the BBL method rather than their medication to overcome their attacks. Thirty-eight (73%) discontinued their medication as soon as they commenced the BBL method. Eight (15%) cut down their medication after three to four days. Steroid medications, however, were an exception. They had to be reduced gradually. The patients were allowed to take their medication in conjunction with the treatment only if they were unable to stop the attack after ten to fifteen minutes with the BBL method. For these cases, medication dosage was reduced by a factor of 2 to 3 and remained sufficient to stop the attack.

THE RESULTS OF THE BBL METHOD

Fifty-two children were observed for twenty-nine to eighty-four days. The results were based on the following criteria:

a. no improvement

b. some improvement (The degree of attacks is lessened together with a considerable reduction in medication.)

c. considerable improvement (cessation of the heavy attacks, slight traces of the disease, or a total disappearance of the symptoms)

The results are listed in Table III.

Table III—Results of the BBL method

Group	Considerable Improvement	Some Improvement	No change	Worse
Hospital	28 (82.4%)	6 (17.6%)	0	0
Ambulatory	15 (83.3%)	3 (16.6%)	0	0
Total	43 (82.7%)	9 (17.3%)	0	0

Forty-three (83%) of the patients showed considerable improvement and nine (17%) showed some improvement. There were no cases showing no improvement. The average period of hospitalization was sixteen days. All the patients with bronchial asthma (52) improved in the first four days. They could breathe freely through the nose, and their coughs and wheezing disappeared. Fifteen experienced "sanogenes" (self-cleansing) reactions, manifesting themselves through nervous excitement, chills, raised temperatures (up to 39°C), headaches, muscular pains, intestinal pains, chest pains, weakness and hypersecretion of mucus. Some experienced appetite loss, nausea, vomiting, thirst, excessive salivation (smelling of their medication), and increased urination and defecation. These reactions lasted from a few hours to two days and happened two to three times. The time in the condition of the patient was relative to the length of the controlled pause.

The clinical observations of the dynamics and the functions of the bronchi were researched simultaneously (using Tiffno tests and the Rait scale). All the patients showed the following results during the first fourteen days of the BBL treatment.

As the control pause increased from ten to forty seconds, so did the concentrations of immunoglobulins A, M, G, and E. Forced expiration volume (Rait's measuring scale) was raised from 36.7 to 173.2 (see Table IV). The acid-alkali balance of the blood normalized (it became less basic), the pCO_2 of the arterial blood increased from 24.6 to 36.3 mmHg. Control pause increased from 2.9 (+/− 0.3) seconds to 31.4 (+/− 4.7) seconds (see Table V).

Table IV—Change in lung capacity with the BBL treatment

State of illness	Number	Start point	40 mins	Time in days 7	14	30
Severe	14	37 (+/−8)	82 (+/−11)	117 (+/−15)	159 (+/−16)	—
Average	26	76 (+/−8)	121 (+/−8)	161 (+/−18)	173 (+/−10)	139 (+/−9)

Table V—Change in control pause with the BBL treatment

State of illness	Number	Start point	40 mins	Time in days 7	14	30
Severe	14	2.9 (+/−.3)	12.4 (+/−1.4)	28.0 (+/−4.9)	24.5 (+/−4.5)	31.4 (+/−4.7)
Average	26	5.4 (+/−.7)	12.5 (+/−1.8)	24.0 (+/−3.9)	28.3 (+/−6.4)	31.4 (+/−4.7)

Patients with severe cases of asthma increased their lung capacities by 27 percent; the allergic resistance increased by 33 percent (see Table VI).

Table VI—Change in lung capacity (LC), allergic resistance (AR), and expiration speed (ES) with the BBL treatment

State of illness	Number	Time Start LC	AR	ES	14 days LC	AR	ES
Severe	8	39.2	29.4	22.1	66.2	62.0	72.3
Average	15	55.3	48.0	51.0	80.0	78.3	85.3

CONCLUSION

1. The BBL method, as suggested by Dr. Buteyko, helps to decrease the number and severity of attacks as well as the dosage of medication.
2. As a result of this therapy, the indicators of acid-alkali balance and lung ventilation improved.
3. The method may be taught to children from three years of age up, either in hospital or as outpatients.
4. This method is endured by children of any age over three.
5. This method is most effective in acute periods of bronchial asthma in very ill patients.

3

A SUMMARY OF THE AUSTRALIAN
BUTEYKO ASTHMA TRIAL

A semiblind, randomized study trial comparing the effects of the Buteyko breathing technique with a placebo breathing technique was funded by the Australian Association of Asthma Foundations.

It was conducted at the Mater Hospital in Brisbane and was designed and monitored by some of Australia's foremost medical asthma specialists.

Severe-asthma sufferers were randomly allocated into either the Buteyko group or the placebo group. This was done in such a way as to result in statistically equal groups in terms of asthma severity and drug usage.

The Buteyko group (nineteen people) was taught Buteyko; the placebo group (twenty people) was given general asthma education, relaxation exercises, and was taught nonhyperventilation breathing exercises (abdominal breathing).

Patients kept diary cards at home, scoring symptoms (3 =

maximal symptoms; 0 = no symptoms), PEF, and medication usage.

Please note that all measurements are statistically significant unless otherwise stated.

RESULTS AT SIX WEEKS

Beta-agonist use

Buteyko group decreased average agonist use by 90.1 percent (from 1235ug to 134ug).
Placebo group decreased average agonist use by 5 percent (from 1029ug to 978ug).

Inhaled-steroid use

Buteyko group average inhaled-steroid use fell 12.5 percent (from 1893ug to 1656ug).
Placebo group average inhaled-steroid use remained statistically the same (at 1450ug to 1551ug).

Diary card symptom scores

Buteyko group decreased symptoms score by 50 percent.
Placebo group decreased symptoms score by 15 percent.

Quality of life score—impact of asthma on patient lives

Dimensions measured were breathlessness, mood, impact on social activity, concern for the future.
Buteyko group—54 percent improvement, better in all dimensions.
Placebo group—24 percent worsening.

SUMMARY AT SIX WEEKS

After six weeks Buteyko subjects used 90 percent less beta-agonist (relief medication), felt substantially better in terms of breathlessness, mood, social activity, and concerns about the future; had fewer symptoms; and as a group used less inhaled steroids.

RESULTS AT THREE MONTHS

Beta-agonist use

Buteyko group had maintained decreased average use by 90 percent.
Placebo group had increased average use by 9 percent.

Inhaled-steroid use

Buteyko group had decreased average use by 49 percent.
Placebo group was statistically the same as before the trial.

Diary card symptom scores

Buteyko group—71 percent improvement.
Placebo group—14 percent improvement.

Quality of life scores

Buteyko group had significant improvement that was still maintained at eight months.

FOLLOW-UP AT EIGHT MONTHS

At eight months the decrease in beta-agonist use in the Buteyko group had been maintained.

DISCUSSION

This study showed that a group of severe asthmatics (averaging over twelve puffs of relief medication) were able to reduce their medication to an average of just over one puff per day, simply by learning a different model for breathing. As well as reduced relief medication, the need for steroids was also significantly reduced. This is combined with massively reduced symptoms and greatly improved quality of life.

In this trial it was also attempted to monitor changes in CO_2 levels, changes in peak expiratory flow levels, and minute volume levels. Because of the relatively small sample size, the only statistically significant change among these measures of lung function was minute volume. Minute volume is an objective measure of the volume of air breathed at rest in one minute while stable. It is a consistent measure of the degree of hyperventilation of the patient. The Buteyko group average minute volume dropped from 14.0 + 6.5 liters to 9.6 + 3.1 liters, which is a significant drop when compared to the placebo group. This change is exactly as predicted by the Buteyko theory, which states that a reduction in hyperventilation will result in reduction in symptoms of asthma and hay fever. (Correlation was found between the relative reduction in beta-agonist use in the Buteyko group and the relative reduction in minute volume, $r = 0.51$, $p = 0.4$.)

This trial summary is taken from *The Buteyko Manual* by James Hooper, Buteyko Practitioner, Townsville, Australia. Phone: (61) 77-255160, Fax: (61) 77-255578; Email: hooper @ultra.net.au. *The Buteyko Manual* (ISBN: 0-646-32419-5) is published by Instep International Press, 1996.

GLOSSARY

Albuterol–a commonly prescribed bronchodilator.

Bronchial–of or relating to the lungs.

Bronchodilator–a drug which dilates the bronchial tubes, apparently facilitating breathing.

Bronchospasm–the involuntary contraction of the bronchial tubes, which is part of the mechanism of an asthma attack.

Control pause–the length of time you can hold your breath after breathing out and not feel the need to breathe again. An ideal control pause is sixty seconds; a control pause of fifteen or below indicates serious and chronic asthma.

Cromolyn–a drug first marketed in the 1960s. It failed to achieve the "miracle cure" status originally claimed for it, but is still commonly prescribed for children suffering from asthma.

Hyperventilation–overbreathing, that is, taking in more air than the internationally recognized physiological norm. It is a fundamental principle of Dr. Buteyko's teaching that many diseases— and all forms of asthma—are caused by hyperventilation.

Nebulizer–a method of administering bronchodilating drugs that is as much as fifty times more intense than the familiar inhaler.

Peak flow meter–a device used in conventional medicine to measure "force-expiration," i.e., the amount of air you can blow out in one attempt.

Reliever medicine–drug that relieves symptoms (such as bronchospasm in asthma) without attempting to prevent the disease.

Steroid–a drug which is chemically similar to a natural hormone and which is commonly prescribed as an anti-inflammatory. Steroids are an important preventive treatment for asthma and can be given intravenously as an emergency treatment during an asthma attack.

REFERENCES

Adam, James. 1926. *Asthma and Its Radical Treatment*. London: Kimpton.

Ameisen, Dr. Paul J. 1997. *Every Breath You Take*. Sydney, Aust.: Lansdowne Publishing.

Benson, R., and F. Perlman. 1948. Clinical effects of epinephrine by inhalation. *Journal of Allergy* 19: 129–40.

Bhagat, R., et al. 1996. Salbutamol-induced increased airway responsiveness to allergen and reduced protein versus methacholine: dose response. *Journal of Allergy & Clinical Immunology* 1, part 1.

Blauw, G., and R. Westendrop. 1995. Asthma Deaths in New Zealand: Whodunnit? *Lancet* 345: 2–3.

Bowler, S., A. Green, C. Mitchell, and T. Graham. Buteyko breathing in asthma: a controlled trial. Mater Hospital, South Brisbane, Queensland (paper available from Dr. S. Bowler, Mater Hospital, South Brisbane, Queensland 4101, Australia).

Brisco, Paula. 1997. *Asthma: Questions You Have, Answers You Need*. London: Thorsons.

British Medical Association. 1950. *Fifty Years of Medicine*. London.

Burney, P. G. J. 1991. Strategy for Asthma. *British Medical Journal* 303: 571–73.

Christian, H. A., and J. Mackenzie, eds. 1932. *The Oxford Medicine*. Oxford: Oxford University Press.

Clarke, P. S. 1971. Effect of disodium cromoglycate on exacerbations of asthma produced by hyperventilation. *British Medical Journal* 1: 317–19.

——— 1980. Asthma hyperventilation and emotion. *Australian Family Physician* 9, October.

Cochrane, et al. 1975. A survey of asthma mortality in patients between ages 35 and 64 in the Greater London hospitals. *Thorax*: 30.

Coke, F. 1932. *Asthma*. Bristol: Wright & Sons.

Conybeare, J. J. 1929. *A Textbook of Medicine*. Edinburgh: Livingstone.

Corrigan, C. 1992. Mechanism of glucocorticoid action in asthma; too little too late. *Clin. Exp. Allergy* 22: 315–17.

Crane, J., N. Pearce, A. Flatt et al. 1989. Prescribed fenosterol and death from asthma in New Zealand 1981–1983: a case control study. *Lancet* 1: 917–22.

Donnell, P. 1991. Exercise-induced asthma: the protective role of CO_2 during swimming. *Lancet* 337: 179–80.

Douthwaite, A. H. *The Treatment of Asthma*. London: H. K. Lewis.

Downes, S. 1995. Article from *Airways*, summarized in The beta agonist debate: new insights. *The Asthma Welfarer* (vi): 29, no. 1: 3.

Drinkwater, H. *Fifty Years of Medical Progress (1873–1922)*. London.

Folgering, H., and A. Snik. 1988. Hyperventilation syndrome and muscle fatigue. *Journal of Psychosomatic Research* 32.

Gayrard, P., J. Orehek, C. Grimaud, and J. Charpin. 1975. Bronchoconstrictor effects of a deep inspiration in patients with asthma. *American Review of Respiratory Diseases* 111: 433–39.

Gould, Donald. *The Medical Mafia*. London: Faber.

Graham, T. Self-management of asthma through normalization of breathing. The role of breathing therapy. Paper distributed to delegates at National Asthma Conference, Brisbane, Australia, October 1996. Available through the Asthma Foundation of Queensland.

Haldane, J. S. 1905. The absorption and dissociation of CO_2 by human blood. *Journal of Physiology*.

——— 1905. The regulation of the lung-ventilation. *Journal of Physiology* 5:32.

——— 1917. Organism and environment as illustrated by the physiology of breathing.

Haldane, J. S., and J. Priestley. 1935. *Respiration*.

Hall, Percy. 1930. *Asthma and Its Treatments*. London: Heinemann.

Herxheimer, Herbert G. J. 1952. *The Management of Bronchial Asthma.* London: Butterworth.

Hibbert, G., and D. Pilsbury. 1988. Demonstration and treatment of hyperventilation causing asthma. *British Journal of Psychiatry* 53: 687–89.

Hopkins, A. 1995. *Epilepsy.* London: Arnold

Hormbrey, J., et al. 1988. CO_2 response and patterns of breathing in patients with symptomatic hyperventilation compared to asthmatic and normal subjects. *European Respiratory Journal* 1: 846–52.

Illich, Ivan. 1991. *Limits to Medicine.* London: Penguin.

———— 1998. *Medical Nemesis: The Exploitation of Health.* London: Random House.

Innocenti, Dr. 1986. "Chronic Hyperventilation" in *Text Book for Physiotherapists.* London.

Lane, Donald J. 1996. *Asthma: The Facts.* 3rd ed. Oxford: Oxford University Press.

Lask, Aaron. *Asthma: Attitude and Milieu.* Tavistock Publications.

Lasko, K. A. *The Great Billion Dollar Medical Swindle.*

Lewis, K. H., and J. B. L. Howell. 1986. Definition of the HVS. *Bulletin of European Physiopathology and Respiration* 22: 201.

Medical Sciences Bulletin. June 1994. Serevent: Long-acting inhaler for asthma. Pharmaceutical Information Associates Ltd.

Mitchell, C., S. Bowler, and Buteyko (Aust.) P/L. Agreement for Buteyko Trial. November 1994.

National Asthma Campaign, Melbourne. 1993. *Asthma Management Handbook.*

Naughton, M., D. Benard, R. Rutherford, and T. Bradley. 1994. Effect of continuous positive airway pressure on central sleep apnea and nocturnal PCO_2 in heart failure. *American Journal of Critical Care Medicine* 1509, 1598–1604.

New England Journal of Medicine quoted in *The Asthma Welfarer.* 1995. 29: 1, 3.

O'Donnell, S. The drug therapy of asthma—what are the outstanding questions? Paper presented at National Asthma Conference, Brisbane, October 1996.

Pearce, N., R. Beasley, J. Crane et al. 1995. End of the New Zealand asthma mortality epidemic. *Lancet* 345: 41–44.

Royal Society of Medicine. 1984. *Nocturnal Asthma.* London.

Salter, Henry Hyde. 1860. *Asthma: Its Pathology and Treatment.* Edinburgh: Churchill.

Sears, M., et al. 1987. 75 deaths in asthmatics prescribed home nebulizers. *British Medical Journal,* 294.

Sears, M., D. Taylor, C. Print et al. 1993. Regular inhaled salbutamol may exacerbate bronchial inflammation in patients with mild asthma. *Thorax* 48: 1060.

Selroos, O., et al. 1988. Effect of early vs late intervention with inhaled corticosteroids in asthma. *Chest* 108: 1228–34.

Serafini, U. 1992. Can fatal asthma be prevented?—A personal view. *Clin. Exp. Allergy* 22: 576–88.

Speizer et al. 1968. Observations on recent increase in mortality from asthma. *British Medical Journal* 1.

——— 1986. Investigation into use of drugs preceding death from asthma. *British Medical Journal* 1.

Tobin, M. J. et al. 1963. Breathing patterns. Diseased subjects. *Chest* 84: 287–94.

Van den Elshout, F., J. van Herwaarden, and H. Folgering. 1991. Effects of hypercapnia and hypocapnia on respiratory resistance in normal and asthmatic subject. *Thorax* 46: 28–32.

West, B. 1990. *Respiratory Physiology.* 4th ed., Williams & Wilkins.

Wilbur, R. L. 1938. *The March of Medicine.* Connecticut: Stamford University Press.

Woolcock, A. J., and J. Read. 1965. Improvement in asthma not reflected in forced expiratory volume. *Lancet* 2: 1323.

Youngson, Dr. Robert. 1995. *Living with Asthma.* London: Sheldon Press.

INDEX

ABOUT THE AUTHOR

Alexander (Sasha) Stalmatski was trained by Dr. Buteyko and worked with him in Russia for fourteen years. He brought the Breath Connection to the West in 1990, working in Australia for six years. During this time, he treated about six thousand asthmatics and trained forty-five Buteyko practitioners. Now based at the Hale Clinic in London, he represents Dr. Buteyko and his methods outside Russia.

Information about Breath Connection workshops can be found at the Hale Clinic website: www.haleclinic.com, emailing at admin@haleclinic.com, or by calling 1 (800) 259-4044.